A Programing Contingency Analysis of Mental Health

A Programing Contingency Analysis of Mental Health presents Dr. Israel Goldiamond's reflections on various ways we formulate behavioral and emotional problems, most often in traditional terms of mental health disorders, mental diseases or illnesses, psychopathological disorders, and so on – what he calls a pathological orientation. Here, Goldiamond argues for a groundbreaking alternative view from the vantage point of radical behaviorism.

The book begins by discussing contingency relations between behavior and its past and present consequences, along with other environmental events. It reminds us that this approach sits comfortably alongside other consequential systems in the social and biological sciences, particularly decision theory and evolution. This behaviorist system regards most important human behaviors as being emitted rather than stimulus-elicited. Described are some of the diverse origins of behavior, including the effects of environmental consequences and the programing procedures of social and cultural inheritance. The exposition includes decision matrices that rationalize some of the programed patterns and the accompanying thoughts and emotions commonly found in mental illness. As a result of this nonlinear contingency analysis, such patterns may be considered adaptive rather than maladaptive. The book describes programs based on those matrices and outlines how they might be applied to mitigate any problems or costs associated with those patterns. It concludes by moving from individual analysis to social analysis, with particular reference to some societal contingencies that may maintain the pathological orientation and others that might shift our gaze in the direction proposed here.

Alongside Dr. Goldiamond's original work, this volume features a new introduction from Dr. Paul Thomas Andronis and Dr. T. V. Joe Layng, as well as an article tracing the history of the nonlinear thinking of Dr. Goldiamond, first published in *The Behavior Analyst*. It will be a must-read for anyone working in the analysis of and clinical intervention in problems associated with mental health, or those more generally interested in the work of Israel Goldiamond.

Israel Goldiamond, a pioneer in the field of behavioral psychology, was a professor in psychiatry, behavior sciences (biopsychology), and medicine (committee on nutrition and nutritional biology) and Director of the Behavior Analysis Research Laboratory at the University of Chicago. Goldiamond was a fellow of both the American Association for the Advancement of Science and the American Psychological Association, and he served as the international president for the Association for Behavior Analysis from 1977 to 1978.

Behavior Science

Series Editor: The Association for Behavior Analysis International

Applied Behavior Science in Organizations: Consilience of Historical and Emerging Trends in Organizational Behavior Management
Edited by Ramona A. Houmanfar, Mitch Fryling & Mark P. Alavosius

A Programing Contingency Analysis of Mental Health
Israel Goldiamond

For more information about this series, please visit: www.routledge.com/Behavior-Science/book-series/ABAI

A Programing Contingency Analysis of Mental Health

Israel Goldiamond

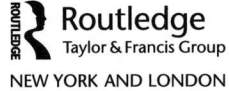

Routledge
Taylor & Francis Group

NEW YORK AND LONDON

Cover image: © Martin Burch

First published 2022
by Routledge
605 Third Avenue, New York, NY 10158

and by Routledge
2 Park Square, Milton Park, Abingdon, Oxon, OX14 4RN

Routledge is an imprint of the Taylor & Francis Group, an informa business

© 2022 ABAI

Library of Congress Cataloging-in-Publication Data
A catalog record for this title has been requested

ISBN: 9781032196237 (hbk)
ISBN: 9781032196220 (pbk)
ISBN: 9781003260103 (ebk)

DOI: 10.4324/9781003260103

Typeset in Minion Pro
by Newgen Publishing UK

Contents

Foreword

Paul Thomas Andronis and T. V. Joe Layng

When do we dare to point to a work in psychology as a "tour-de-force"? Without any hesitation, this can be said of Israel Goldiamond's *A Programing Contingency Analysis of Mental Health*. The argument Goldiamond makes in this short book is built carefully, step by step – from the philosophical underpinnings of the science of behavior, to societal contingencies giving rise to traditional formulations of mental illness and practices derived therefrom – culminating in an alternative radical behaviorist (and highly humanistic) approach to clinical analysis and treatment. This analysis is grounded equally in the experimental analysis of behavior and careful observation of *in vivo* contingencies at work in free-ranging human behavior observed in the clinic. The force of the argument rests in its logic, coherence, and overarching view that all human activity runs through a river of contingencies. It felt as though most of these ideas were ahead of the times when they were first presented. We suggest that in many ways they still are.

This is not a "how to" book. For those interested in the clinical applications of the approach pioneered by Goldiamond and his students, there are other resources, such as the recently published *Nonlinear Contingency Analysis: Going Beyond Behavior and Cognition in Clinical Practice*. This is, instead, an analysis of the contingencies responsible for patterns often requiring such intervention, and the societal contingencies that govern how such patterns are viewed.

An earlier, briefer version of this book was originally delivered on May 15, 1978, as the Presidential Address to the 4th Annual Convention of the Midwest Association for Behavior Analysis (MABA was the progenitor to ABAI), held in Chicago, IL, at the Blackstone Hotel. The talk went well beyond its allocated hour. The MABA talk occasioned what we recall as mixed reactions. Some audience members were excited by its scope, depth, and the revealing connections it made among conceptual issues, as evidenced by many animated discussions that followed and continued through dinner and after. A few others mainly groused about its length. The manuscript was later revised and expanded and was to appear as a chapter in a book on philosophy and medicine. The length became an issue during the editorial process, and Goldiamond withdrew it from the book. Since its most recent version, authored in 1983, the paper has been reedited for minor stylistic matters, more contemporary terminology where necessary, and a few added references. But its present form remains substantively unchanged from the original version and as potentially influential as it should have been at the start.

In 1934, Jakob von Uexküll wrote an impactful treatise titled "A Stroll Through the Worlds of Animals and Men." In it, he described how the world as perceived by different organisms was indeed quite distinctive for each organism. Goldiamond lived in and distinctively saw a world of behavioral contingencies. He not only spoke about contingencies but also lived them and perceived them with a unique clarity. As newly minted grad students in Goldiamond's lab at the University of Chicago, what we heard and later read was a clearly articulated and orderly tour of previously encountered ideas, contingency analyses, and examples familiar to us from his course lectures, from regular free-for-all discussions during weekly lab meetings, and from daily informal conversations walking with him the half-mile between his home and the lab, or the mile each way between our lab and the main campus. Many of these ideas had come up in relation to ongoing human and animal experiments in our lab, current clinical cases being managed by our various staff members, sharp questions posed by students in his courses, and recently published work that had caught the attention of someone in our group. At other times, the ideas were occasioned by data or concepts from other fields altogether (like evolutionary/developmental biology, physics, political science, economics, and so on) that Goldiamond "just happened to come across" during his customary browsing through broad swaths of scholarly literature. In his view, all these matters were interrelated – and all were amenable to analysis of the contingencies that gave rise to them.

Goldiamond, fondly known to us as Izzy, routinely assimilated these new materials and, through careful formal analysis, brought them into accord with what he already knew. His published works, appearing in the experimental, clinical, instructional, legal, and theoretical literatures, comprise a continuous "fossil record" of the systematic evolution of his thinking (see the appendix of this book for a detailed narrative of the paths his work took).

We recently rediscovered an unpublished manuscript of Izzy's (titled "Contingencies of Schizophrenia") that slightly predates the present work. In it, he describes several kinds of contingency relations he encountered many times over in his psychiatric casework, many of which are described in the current book. This initial formulation was undoubtedly influenced, at least in part, by a long discussion that occurred in a lab meeting, occasioned by a pair of (then) recent popular books on transactional analysis, *I'm Okay, You're Okay* (Harris) and *Games People Play* (Berne), brought to our attention by one of our clinical postdocs. At first, a few of us "committed" radical behaviorists dismissed the books as just pop psychology, of no real interest, but... Goldiamond then proceeded to describe for us the derivation of this popular form of transactional analysis from its empirical roots in cultural anthropology and quickly pointed out that the transactions described could be viewed in terms of the interlocking social contingencies they represented. A couple of weeks later, he began dropping descriptions of some of these contingencies into his classroom lectures, using terms like "blackmail contingencies," "day in the sun contingencies," "legitimating contingencies," "junk behavior," and so on, which appeared with more formal exposition in the manuscript on schizophrenia and subsequently in the present book on contingencies of mental health.

This anecdote is meant to illustrate what made Izzy's thinking and tutelage so valuable and engaging. First, he rarely dismissed any matter out of hand because it violated or ignored some behaviorist orthodoxy. Smart people could be mistaken or plainly wrong, but there was almost always some kernel of discernable stimulus control that might point the way to something more important or useful in their work. He always took the time to explore such options. He was always "constructional" and contingency-analytic in his thinking, even when following the wrong turns or missteps of other scholars. Second, with the wheels of his wheelchair planted firmly, one pair on scientific grounds and the other in applied settings, he always looked for ways to communicate dense technical matters in language that laypersons (and students) could readily comprehend, using words like "occasion" for antecedents or discriminative stimuli or the use of "blackmail" to describe one form of negative reinforcement contingencies at work in certain social arrangements, and so on. Though his professional publications can be challenging reads for some, the people who sought help came prepared with their own potent vocabularies, and Goldiamond tried to make contact with them as much as possible on their own terms.

This brings us to a final point, namely, his concern with identifying or establishing a common vocabulary as part of his larger vision that effective change procedures arose from meticulous programing of contingencies. In his expanded model of the operant paradigm, particularly when describing behavior change, the "program" was included as an explicit variable. By program, he meant a systematic series of changes in occasions for behavior and in the criteria for producing contingent consequences, leading from a subject's entry repertoire to some targeted outcome. A person's history, so central to much clinical lore, he treated as a retrospective attempt to identify past programs that led to the person's current status. Together, history and the program pointed the way ahead. This book is one outcome of the program that made Goldiamond's contributions so unique.

1

Introduction

Mental illness is presently defined in a variety of ways. It is defined as a pathology of thought or affect that may or may not be manifest in behavior. It may be defined in terms of ways of relating to the environment. Agreement is not universal. Mental illness, for example is considered to be a myth (Szasz, 1961), a label of deviance applied by a society that may thereby exacerbate the problem (Becker, 1963; Scheff, 1966), a "disjunction between two persons," one of whom is considered sane (Laing, 1969 p. 37). Where the patterns are interpreted to indicate pathology, the pathology may be defined biologically, in organic or genetic terms (cf. Rosenthal, 1970) or may be defined in terms of conditioned behavior disorders (cf. Rachman and Teasdale, 1969), in addition to the more traditional psychodynamic and other psychiatric formulations, which have been in transition since, at least, Kraepelin's formulations.

These differences in interpretation represent, to a considerable extent, serious efforts to understand the patterns, to intervene when problems are perceived, and to relate intervention and understanding so that one or both may be advanced. Accordingly, the differences in interpretation relate to differences in professional intervention – and social consequences: for an example, we need not go so far afield as Nazi Germany but can reflect on this country's "eugenic sterilization laws which were passed … [for] eventual elimination of insanity and feeblemindedness," starting in 1907, and on the books of twenty-seven states in 1968 (Paul, 1968, pp. 77–78). The fact that such an approach is rationalized by a genetic model does not, of course, associate present supporters of such models with such interventions but does demonstrate the close relation between theory and practice in this field.

The fact that social institutions have been established for understanding, intervention, and training in this field suggests that its phenomena may not be trivial. And the fact that there is widespread involvement in the services offered suggests that the maintaining variables may be widespread. Accordingly, the study of the phenomena of mental illness and of the circumstances surrounding it may make contributions that extend beyond this special field.

The present discussion will focus on an analysis of these issues from the vantage point of radical behaviorism (Skinner, 1974), to be defined shortly. I shall focus, in part, on the relations between behavior and its past and present consequences and other environmental events. Since this system is generally unknown except, perhaps, in rumor, I shall first spell out the system and clarify its position on events such as emotion and thought. I shall relate this system to other consequential systems in the social and biological sciences, namely, decision theory and evolution. A point-by-point correspondence between evolutionary theory and radical behaviorism will be noted, with special attention given to the parallel between breeding and behavior-programing. Since the system considers behavior to be emitted

DOI: 10.4324/9781003260103-1

rather than stimulus-elicited, I shall next consider the diverse origins of behavior and discuss the effects of environmental consequences and of the programing procedures of social and cultural inheritance upon such diverse behaviors. In the course of this analysis, some decision matrices that rationalize certain programed patterns found in mental illness will be presented, along with programs that might be applied. Finally, I shall move from individual analysis to social analysis with particular reference to some societal consequences that may maintain the pathological ideology; other possibilities will be noted.

The analytic system to be used

2.1 CONFUSIONS BETWEEN FORMULATIONS

The term *behavior analysis* will be used here in the context of *radical behaviorism*, a term applied by B. F. Skinner (1945, 1974) to distinguish it from more traditional behaviorisms. The distinction is an important one. Attacks upon Skinner and his followers often cite the philosophy of the latter (Day, 1969) and the scientific paradigms they employ.[1] In part, the confusion stems from the existence of at least two different underlying philosophies of and approaches in a science of behavior. These often use similar terms to study similar topics in different ways. In addition, two different sets of learning formulations similarly confuse differences between them. These two sets of differences intersect in part.

These differences in psychologies are of interest to others. Any definitions of mental health and mental illness must include a behavioral component. The general stance taken toward behavior must affect the specific concepts it helps to define. Further, an interesting paradox will become evident. Prevailing theories (and less systematic understandings) of mental health often explicitly reject the philosophic stances they associate with behaviorism. However, in so doing, they implicitly follow assumptions associated with behaviorism – of one kind, rather than another. Acceptance or rejection of these assumptions is among the differences between the behaviorisms.

One of my purposes here is to make explicit these assumptions and their major implications for theory and practice in mental health/illness. In so doing, it will be necessary to distinguish between the different uses of similar terms. The occurrence of this confusion has an understandable historical base that is irrelevant to the discussion. Accordingly, wherever necessary, I shall attempt to substitute terms that more closely approximate common usage; in such cases, technical jargon will be relegated to endnotes. Generally, my discussions of the philosophies and learning formulations will be limited to their relevance to the mental health issue under consideration.

2.2 REACTIVE AND CONSEQUENTIAL RELATIONS

Rather than opening with distinctions in the philosophies, I shall open with the learning formulations whose differences contributed to the philosophies. These learning formulations may be designated as the *reactive* and the *consequential*.[2] The former conceptualizes behavior in terms of its antecedent stimuli and explains behavior as a response (or reaction) to such

DOI: 10.4324/9781003260103-2

events. The latter conceptualizes behavior in terms of its effects on the environment and explains behavior through the consequences it produces. The differences are quite meaningful in the psychological laboratory. In the former case, presentation of a stimulus will elicit the behavior, as in a reflex. In the latter case, it is the occurrence of the behavior that produces the stimulus, as in purchase of a commodity.

These differences reflect meaningful distinctions in other disciplines and approaches. This will be evident if we attempt to explain a patient's violent outburst in a psychiatric ward. The observed events occur in the following older: an attendant informs a patient that as long as the patient smokes, the attendant will avoid the fumes by sitting elsewhere. The patient glares at the attendant and continues to smoke. Shortly thereafter, at the scheduled time, the head nurse enters the ward. The patient begins to scream, crawls and writhes on the floor, and is finally quieted. At the next day's staff meeting, the head nurse accuses the attendant of insensitivity and holds him responsible for an outbreak that set the patient back.

If we state that the patient's outburst was caused (precipitated) by the attendant's remarks, we are adopting the *linear causality* of the reactive position. In those terms, the attendant's provocation is the stimulus (*L.*, to goad), and the patient's outburst is the response (reaction). We can restrict ourselves to observables and a simple stimulus→response relation. We can infer an internal emotion as a mediating term or condition and consider a more complex stimulus→emotion→response relation. The attendant's remarks elicited resentment and rage that elicited (or emerged as) the outburst. The conventional terminology is illustrative: the patient "acted out," i.e., an *inner* response emerged or became a stimulus for an *outer* response. As is evident, the chain of reasoning is not restricted to the conditioning laboratory nor to observables. The disproportionality of the response to the stimulus arousing it is an "overreaction," and it is this *abnormality* (in the literal sense) that suggests the existence of pathology. At the least, the behavior is maladaptive or disturbed.

If we state that the patient's outburst, by clearly bringing to the attention of the head nurse the attendant's slight, is governed by the retribution the outburst is likely to bring on the attendant, we are adopting the stance of the consequential position. As stated here, the patient's outburst is governed by consequences it may produce at a later time. It is not governed by linear antecedents. Causality flows *away* from behavior, rather than toward it. We can restrict our statement to observables and an occasion- (when)-behavior→consequence relation, or an occasion (when) an *if*-behavior→, *then* consequence relation holds. We can infer concomitant internal intent: to get even←I'll act up, or I'll act up→(to) get even, but such inference is not necessary for the observable relation to hold. That such patterns do occur repeatedly without the patient having figured out the relations in advance, or at all, is suggested by the existence of concepts such as unconscious motivation. As is evident, the chain of reasoning is not restricted to the learning laboratory nor to observables. Presumably, yet another consequence is that the rebuke may serve to keep the attendant in line. Such retributive manipulation, while disturbing to the staff and eventually to the patient, is certainly neither abnormal nor unprecedented.[3] Indeed, it may imply rather finely honed social skills on the part of the patient. At the least, the behavior is adaptive, albeit disturbing.

The two learning formulations, when extended to this situation, speak of different implications for mental illness and different approaches to the behaviors involved. The formulations may be considered to be laboratory-derived examples of different types of reasoning that find more general use. Comparison of systems whose terms tend to be defined explicitly, i.e., laboratory-based systems, may help to understand related systems whose differing implications for mental health may have been obscured by their greater reliance on implicit and less precisely stated terms.

2.2.1 The reactive formulation

As noted, in the reactive formulation, behavior is conceptualized in terms of its antecedent stimuli. Hence the designation, S→R behaviorism, and hence the very terms themselves. The behavior is the *response* (R) to a *stimulus* (S), or stimuli. That the response is a behavioral reaction to an action is implied by the accepted designation for the time-interval between a stimulus and its response, namely, *reaction time*. Stimuli elicit behavior in a linearly causal manner. The S→R relationship, of course, is conditional upon other circumstances. These can include present arrangements and past associations with other stimuli, as in those present relations derived from earlier conditioning.[4]

Classical mentalist approaches reject the automaticity implied. Nevertheless, mediation between S and R through (mental) image or affect (M) often simply adds a mediating term. Such mediation preserves the linear causality noted, namely, S→M→R: the *parents' appearance* (after an absence) so *angered* (upset) the child that a *tantrum* was produced. Linearity is also often found in formulations that impose organic mediation: the S→O→R models. Indeed, Pavlov borrowed the term *reflex* from physiology to designate the relation whose clarification is associated with him.

2.2.2 Consequential relations

As systematized by Skinner (1969, p. 7), the basic building block here is a "three-term contingency." As noted, upon certain *occasions*, the critical *stimulus* follows upon (is produced by) *behavior*: Oc-(S→R) or, stated temporally, Oc-(B→S).[5] Behavior is *not* a response (reaction) to a stimulus. Rather, the stimulus is the *effect* or consequence of behavior.[6] It is the importance of that consequence, and its occurrence *contingent* on behavior, that will govern the likelihood of the behavior when the occasion for the (B→S) relation occurs. An occasion–behavior relation may emerge, Oc-B, but the occasioning events neither elicit nor cause behavior. The relationship between concluding grace and eating (an Oc-B relation) differs from the relationship between the loaded food tray and salivation (an S→R relation). There is actually a fourth element in the consequential relation, and that is the *interrelation* between the terms, which enter into the precise definition of the contingency, e.g., the *schedule*; on occasion X, each delivery of a consequence is contingent on every second occurrence of behavior, upon every fifth, etc., in any of a variety of ratios that are fixed or that vary around an average (as in a slot machine); the consequence is contingent on behavior at a fixed time interval since the last delivery or at variable intervals. Other schedules are possible that have profound effects on behavior, as will be noted.[7]

Classical mentalist approaches also reject the automaticity implied here. Mediating terms express anticipation, expectation, purpose, and volition, among others. However, in contrast to its effects in the reactive formulation, use of such terms does more than simply add a mediating term. It often sets up processes that are independent of the consequence and render it unnecessary. Further, *it imposes the simple linear causality found in reactive formulations upon a system that logically relates events otherwise*. Rather than Oc-(B→S), e.g., when a parent is present, this child's tantrums are maintained by the ensuing attention; the statement becomes Oc-M→B, *viz* when a parent is present, the child's anticipation (of becoming the center of attention) produces a tantrum. It is difficult to distinguish this drastic revision of the three-term contingency from the formal mediational statement of the reactive formulation, namely, S→M→R.[8]

Traditional mentalist approaches have, on the one hand, denounced the simplicity of the reactive conditioning model and have, on the other, so accepted its simple statement of linear causality as to impose it on a system that relates events differently.

2.3 TRADITIONAL AND RADICAL BEHAVIORISM

Intersecting the reactive and consequential approaches are several organized strategies of analyzing behavior and its relation to other events. Skinner (1974), in his first chapter (pp. 9–20), singles out structuralism, methodological behaviorism, and radical behaviorism. Developmentalism, mentalism, and physicalism are defined in passing.[9] I have noted linear similarities between mentalist, physicalist (organic), and classical behaviorist approaches. To the extent that other approaches share linear causality, they provide formally equivalent terms to explain behavior, despite other differences assigned to these terms. I shall designate those approaches that share linear causality as *traditional approaches*. I shall define *traditional behaviorism* as the behaviorist subset of the traditional approaches.[10] They differ from mentalism in adhering to operationism, and in other ways. Such differences between the traditional approaches have tended to obscure the importance of their common reliance on linear causality. Accordingly, an examination of traditional behaviorism may have relevance for an analysis of mentalism.

2.3.1 Comparative treatments of motivation

As a case study of differences between traditional and radical approaches to behaviorism, I shall consider the term *motivation of behavior*. The importance of the empirical referents of the term does not have to be spelled out. The term, as stated, is linearly causal with regard to behavior: M→B. The empirical problem, so stated, is how to produce M. In early discussions of traditional behaviorism, the M→B statement was paralleled by D→B, with drive (D) being operationally defined. At least one formulation of drive as used in traditional behaviorism is highly congenial to translation into subjective formulation and has, accordingly, been influential in traditional mentalism.[11] In this formulation, one operation entering into the definition of drive is time since, say, last feeding. The greater the deprivation, the greater the hunger drive (or the level of motivation) for food and the stronger the ensuing behavior relevant to the drive (appetitive behavior) and the setting. When the food is found, the organism will consume it (consummatory behavior).[12] Ingestion of food reduces the time since last feeding and reduces hunger drive and its sequelae. These effects on drive may be defined simply as drive reduction or as satiation. Although operationists do not do so, the temptation to infer the subjective experiences of hunger and satiation is strong, as is the effort to interpret them organically. Hence the search for physiological *correlates* of subjective experiences or states. The formal requirements of linear causality are fulfilled by any of these mediating terms.

Needless to say, behavior can be *activated* by other drives (subjective needs, physiological states), such as security, recognition, or power. All of these formulations permit the question of whether behavior is motivated by drive reduction (relief from tension, etc.) or by drive fulfillment (goal attainment).

The same behavior–environment relations may be considered without reference to a linear formulation of activation of behavior (M→B). In a radical behaviorist formulation, the motivational problem is expressed in terms of making potent (or potentiating) a *contingency component*, either Oc, B, S, their relations, or combinations. Although it is not necessary to deprive an organism to "motivate behavior" (one can manipulate the schedule, for example), deprivation was used in the food example mentioned, and I shall therefore use it here. Deprivation would simply be defined as a procedure (there are others) that affects the potency of the *consequence* component of the contingency. The greater the period of deprivation, the more potent the food consequence and the greater the likelihood of the behavior that produces it, when the occasion for B→S occurs; since the occurrence of this occasion

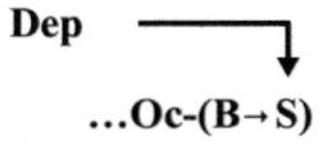

FIGURE 2.1 The form of the relation of deprivation to consequences and behavior

may be contingent on other behavior, the more potent a consequence it will be, and the greater the likelihood of those behaviors that produce it when the occasion for B→S occurs. The same observations are accounted for as before, but there is no reference to drive. The form of the relation of deprivation to consequences and behavior, presented temporally and restricted to "consummatory" behavior, for simplification, can be seen in Figure 2.1.

The form contrasts with the linearity of Dep→Drive→B. Rather than food-deprivation serving to increase hunger drive, or food-ingestion serving to reduce it (B→Dt+l< Dt, where B is ingestion, and t is time), food ingestion serves to decrease the value (reinforcing function, in the operant sense; see note 4) of food. This is a simple statement: if absence of food increases its potency in the contingency, presenting it attenuates its potency. Deprivation and satiation are simply the names of different poles of the same procedure for influencing the potency of a consequence. The simplicity of these statements and the fact that such simplicity is present are both obscured by the imposition of a separate mediating term that is defined independently. One could state that it was this term that occasioned the substitution or addition of subjective or physiological mediators, or both, and that all these make linearity possible as a consequence of such terminological behavior.[13] However, I suspect that a better statement may be that it is the necessity for linear causality (as an outcome of terminologizing) that makes highly likely the behavior of using mediating terms on the occasions when we discuss behavior, in either the theoretical contexts noted or the contexts of the clinic or mental health centers.

The term, drive, is not necessary to at least one formulation; neither is the drive reduction–fulfillment controversy. A topic of equal status is the motivation of behavior. Substituting the potentiation of a contingency, while not solving the empirical problem addressed, offers a different approach by its very formulation. Rather than noting that behavior can be motivated by differing drives, we might note that, just as occasions differ, so will behaviors, consequences, and relations between these, as will the various empirical procedures that make any one or more of these potent. And which of these elements is (or are) critical may differ for the different problems to which mental health is addressed.

Consider gambling, for example. Specification of a gambling drive has posed problems. If its consequence is money, the absence of money that should produce the drive is often the very outcome of the pattern. This might account for the compelling hold of gambling. On the other hand, this is an unusual way for a drive to function. Accordingly, excitement, risk, and a gambling drive itself have served instead. Explanations of their own behavior by gamblers have been used to support these and other explanations. However, it is known that behavior established on variable interval and variable ratio schedules is highly resistant to extinction. Such behavior requires only occasional reinforcement to maintain it. Pigeons, rats, monkeys, and a variety of other animals have continued to behave for inordinately long periods of time, without consequences, after such variable schedules have been in effect for short periods of time. Gambling suggests attention to such *schedules* rather than to *consequences*.[14] Other patterns of mental health problems may require analysis in terms of other contingency elements.

That motivation of *behavior* should be a term of little value to radical behaviorism may upset preconceptions of those who visualize behaviorists as focused narrowly upon behavior. The issue is not narrowness but rather explicitness.

2.4 OPERATIONISM AND INNER EVENTS

In traditional behaviorism, terms are defined operationally, often in a highly sophisticated manner. The mediating term is defined by at least two *independent* operations that converge on the same term (Garner, Hake, and, Eriksen, 1956).[15] Stimulus and response are publicly observable, as are the arrangements, as were the past associations. Accordingly, such nonobservables as emotions and thinking are either excluded or redefined in observable terms that exhaust the definition. Any incorporations into the term of nonobservables are considered surplus or as having "surplus meaning" and are therefore to be rejected. It is probably this feature of traditional behaviorism that mentalists find most unpalatable, since it seems to exclude *the* area of concern: there is more to this world than is found in thy philosophy, Horatio.

Radical behaviorism takes issue with operationism as conventionally defined (see Moore, 1975, for discussion). In contrast to such operationism, the definitions of emotion, thinking, etc., are not exhausted by their convergent operations, nor are they to be so redefined; they are significant terms. In common with mentalism, radical behaviorism distinguishes between public and private events and does not discard the latter. Emotions, thinking, etc., adhere to the latter. However, in contrast to classical mentalism, private terms are not considered as *linearly causal* to behavior. The task is to explain scientifically both sets of events and not to prejudge the issue by making either linearly causal to the other. In this process, procedures that are fruitful in an analysis of public behavior may also be fruitful in an analysis of private events.

2.4.1 Emotions, behavior, and contingencies

A radical behaviorist analysis of emotions may be introduced by resort to Cannon's familiar statement, *I see the bear, I am frightened, therefore I run.* This statement was countered by that of James-Lange, namely, *I see the bear, I run, therefore I am frightened.* This states, in essence, that it is the organic arousal, of which the behavior (running) is a component, that is experienced as fear. The former partakes of the familiar S→M→B form (observable bear stimulus, private fear mediator, observable running behavior). The latter partakes of the familiar linear form S→B→M. The commonly accepted equation of behaviorism with rejection of private events has led to the assumption that behaviorists reject the former formulation and accept the latter. This equation has blinded observers to the fact that it is precisely the former formulation that finds ready acceptance in many clinical areas in psychology and outside it, among many clinical behaviorists, and in writings of some radical behaviorists. Such acceptance is facilitated by (a) the familiar S→M→R form and (b) the ready translation of M into respondent formulation, (c) to which other elements may be added.[16] In all events, it is commonly accepted that emotions are respondents and reactions to the stimuli that elicit them. However, neither the familiar nor the James-Lange nor the respondent formulations consider observable consequences (Skinner, 1971), and I shall consider emotions in such a context, to exemplify a relation between behavior and emotion and observables that accords with radical behaviorism. The example will be in the first person and will include bears, behavior, and emotion to parallel the cited linear form of the two nonconsequential formulations.

As background, we have a cabin in the woods and are out of food. Obtaining food will be a consequence of hunting, and I go out with any rifle. (a) When *I see the bear*, the *consequences* of firing are *obtaining food*, and *I aim and press the trigger*: Oc-(S→B). Emotionally, *I am elated.* However, all my ammunition turns out to be wet, and I produce only a click. The bear growls and comes at me. (b) When *I see the bear* approaching, the consequences of staying are my destruction; I *run* and *maintain my distance* from the pursuing bear: Oc-(S→B) or Oc-(B→S). Emotionally, *I am frightened*. Eventually I am backed up against a cliff. (c) When *I see the bear* approaching, the consequence of impassivity is my mauling; I *threaten* and swing my rifle as a club; *the bear hesitates and keeps its distance*; it is driven off, Oc-(S→B) or Oc-(B→S).[17] Emotionally *I am fighting mad*. In all three cases, given the same occasioning bear, my behaviors change in accord with the shifting consequences of (a) food, (b) escape, and (c) bear withdrawal. In all three cases, given the same occasioning bear, my emotions change in accord with the shifting contingencies. My emotions do not linearly cause my behaviors, nor do my behaviors cause my emotions. *Both emotions and behaviors are governed by the contingencies* and their histories.[18]

In clinical treatment, one can concentrate on affect and its change through a variety of procedures, including chemical or physical interventions; behaviorist- oriented treatments often also concentrate on "counting inners" or on considering emotions as covert responses ("coverants, operants of the mind"). Change in *affect* (by any of these means)→change in behavior. Behaviorist treatments may also view affect as a conditioned response, with change in the conditioned stimulus→a change in affect. On the other hand, one can concentrate on changing the contingencies into which both behavior and affect enter. Many patients who are quite capable of reporting affect do not report the relevant contingencies (they do not *tact* them; cf. Skinner, 1957). The recording of affect, and of circumstances of its experience, can then be used to discover regnant contingencies. Many patients do not report affect. Patients can be *sensitized* to their own emotions as signifying those environmental occasions when behavior is importantly consequential. They can learn to identity these at early stages and act accordingly, while emotion and related contingency are amenable to change (Goldiamond, 1974). Radical behaviorism neither ignores nor defines emotions out of existence. Those forms of psychotherapy that utilize affect to uncover regnant contingencies are in accord with application of radical behaviorism.

I shall resume discussion of emotions when schedule induction is considered.

2.4.2 Awareness and contingencies

There is considerable evidence that contingencies will govern their constituent behaviors whether or not the individual is aware of them. In early laboratory research by Hefferline, Keenan, and Harford (1959), subjects were unaware that environmental change was governed by their behavior and were not even aware of the behavior, but the contingencies governed their behavior. This also held when they were misinformed. Such terms as unconscious and subconscious control imply similarities in clinical experience. And, in the growing bio-feedback literature, the investigator is often the only one who knows the contingencies; the subjects or patients simply try to produce the observable consequence (a light, tone, etc., when organic change meets the criterion set by the investigator), often without knowing just what it is that they are doing, which is effecting change in the consequences. Since it is the presence or absence of contingencies, rather than awareness or nonawareness, that govern their constituent behaviors, the conscious–unconscious *dimension* is irrelevant to the system.

A seminar recently conducted by a psychoanalyst is relevant. He noted that some of his patients changed without having achieved insight into their problems; others who changed had achieved insight. Insight was being implicitly defined as patient ascription of change in a manner congruent with the therapist's ascription of change. Stated otherwise, the patient had learned to use the same system as the therapist in the same way.[19] Such congruences, of course, are achieved by other teachers, politicians, etc., and the common distinction between "insight therapy" and "behavior therapy" is questionable when applied to approaches that provide training of the type described. Be this as it may, other therapists have added that

TABLE 2.1
Possible relations between change, no change, insight, and no insight.

	Insight	*No insight*
Change		
No change		

absence of change can also be accompanied both by presence and absence of insight; given the four possibilities (insight, no insight, by change, no change; see Table 2.1), the change outcome is the critical one both to therapist and patient.

If we define insight in terms of patient ascription in accord with a radical behaviorist ascription, we can relate awareness of contingencies to achievement of outcome in a parallel manner: such change can occur with and without awareness of the relevant contingencies, and such change can be absent with and without such awareness.[20] Which will occur will depend on the conditions and on the program, and there has been experimental investigation of such relations. Where the critical issue is the change, analysis of procedures that can be used to implement it has more than theoretical importance.

Human experience has repeatedly demonstrated that when social and other environmental requirements change, people often persist in the patterns established and governed by preceding requirements, despite the far greater benefits of the new or the high cost of the old. Such persistence has also been demonstrated in operant laboratories when, say, S is unchanged, but the schedule is changed, so that a different pattern of B is required for S. People (and others) may persist in the patterns established and governed by preceding contingencies, despite the greater benefits of the new and the cost of the old. For example, Weiner (1970) changed schedules so that the behavior pattern reinforced under schedule A was disadvantageous at B; the A pattern persisted. If a different schedule, C, was introduced, whether in the sequence ABCBAB, or CAB, or others, patterns appropriate to Schedule B were established – providing patterns appropriate to Schedule C had been established at some preceding time and not otherwise. Producing appropriate behavior required a prior "developmental stage"; when that was absent in the person's history, behavior appropriate to Schedule B was absent (for that series). That gap could be filled by introducing Schedule C, and its introduction constituted effective "therapy."[21] Did awareness (insight) accompany such "therapy"? Weiner (personal communication) reports that no such insight was exhibited. Subjects, when asked to explain differences in their behavior between B periods that were not preceded by C and those which were, reported having "realized" all kinds of events, except the schedules obtaining (see Goldiamond, 1965a, pp. 111–112, for report of similar subjective explanations). What was critical was the *contingency history*.

Indeed, the first (and still elegant) textbook to adopt a radical behaviorist orientation (Keller and Schoenfeld, 1950) devoted a section (pp. 366–371) to such history. The equation of radical behaviorism and ahistory is a misreading.

2.4.3 Instructions, instructional control, and abstraction

If presence of insight, or awareness of contingencies, is irrelevant to control by contingencies, instructions on the nature of the present contingencies or of those to be instituted may facilitate occurrence of the required patterns, or may not, depending on the conditions. Among the critical conditions is whether or not consequences follow upon behavior in accord with instructions about the rule.[22] In marital counseling, for example, one spouse may follow a therapist-suggested rule, but the other spouse may then not reinforce, thereby increasing the likelihood of reinstatement of the partner's original pattern. Parents may behave similarly when the behavior of a child changes. In the laboratory, human *perception* experiments are characterized by (a) presenting the contingency rule in *advance of the occasions*; such advance presentation is designated as *instruction* (G., *Einstellung*). Then (b) the occasions are changed, and corresponding changes in behavior are related to color (form, size, etc.) perception. Human *abstraction* and *concept formation* experiments reverse this (a, b) order. First, (a) the occasions are changed; behaviors in accord with the contingency rule are reinforced and are observed in order to assess when and if (b) behavior in accord with the contingency rule has ensued.[23] Accordingly, control by the contingency rule may emerge *during the presentation* of occasions (Goldiamond, 1966; Skinner, 1966). Such emergence is designated as *abstraction*. Novel presentations, unrelated to those used hitherto, may be presented (to test abstractional control), and the observers may also be asked to state the rule (to test awareness).

In situations outside the laboratory, people often follow rules of conduct relatable to histories of Oc-(B→S) relations; they may then (or may not) explicitly state the induced rules to others and to themselves. As was noted in the discussion of psychotherapy, where change and insight were related in four ways (absence and presence of each), a similar fourfold relation holds in laboratory abstractional control and awareness and also in everyday rule governance of behavior and explicit induction of rules. Whichever of the various fourfold relations hold, all are relatable to a history of Oc-(B→S) relations. Thus, as used here, awareness, insight, and explicit induction of rules are not the epiphenomena to which operationism often assigns them. They do not linearly cause behavior (Oc→Awareness [etc.] →Behavior), nor do behaviors cause awareness, etc. (Oc→Behavior→Awareness). *Both awareness* (insight, explicit induction) *and behavior are governed by the contingencies* and their histories. The fact that one can occasionally precede the other indicates causality no more than it does in emotion and behavior. And, as in different classes of behavior with different histories, they should not be expected to have identical contingency relations. Indeed, instructional control telescopes an extended history of interrelations between both classes of rule governance of behavior.

Where people induce rules, they may instruct their young in them. Such instructions may then function as they do in a perception experiment and govern specific Oc-B relations in advance of their occurrence. In psychotherapy, such instructions provided by the therapist, or rules induced by the patient, may function similarly, with considerable savings. Similarly, presentation of statements of contingencies may be used to induce rules that may then function instructionally. In any case of instruction-governed behavior, if the contingency rule applied is incongruent with the actual Oc-(B→S) arrangements, instructional control may be transient. However, precaution is necessary here. Adventitiously reinforced behavior is likely to be reinforced only intermittently. Related abstractions and instructions induced from these are, because of the adventitious reinforcement attached to behavior under their control, likely to be spurious. Because of the intermittency of the reinforcement, the spurious instructions are likely to be long-lived (cf. Skinner, 1977), despite the simultaneous availability of less spurious instructional and abstractional systems.

Although both require consequences for their control, the type of control over Oc-B relations maintained by instructional or abstractional control differs from the control over B maintained by Oc. For example, one can respond to the same people in different ways. A guide in a museum could name the subject of each portrait on display and do so accurately. The guide could also name the artist, particular painting style, age at time of painting, or other personabilia and could also make a variety of accurate statements about the subject. A guide who accurately describes the painting style of each painting is not likely to have a warm reception from a tour group of psychohistorians. The guide is in "contact with (the)

$$(Inst) \text{ ——— } Set \text{ ——— } (Abst)$$

$$Oc \text{ ——— } (B \to S)$$

FIGURE 2.2 The relation of set control to the stimulus control of behavior

reality" of the paintings but *not of the audience*. If the guide "catches on" and switches to describing interpersonal problems of the artists, such behavior is equally in contact with the paintings but also with audience reinforcement that governed the switch. Abstractional control (attitude) is defined by which of the different categories or stimulus *classes* or *sets* will be applied to each event: naming, style, income, status, clang association (giving a word some of whose sounds resemble those of words typically occasioned by the stimulus), etc. Instructions include telling the guide the stimulus class to apply ahead of time. They might save the speaker grief or time. Stimulus control, as opposed to set control, will be defined by the governance of behavior by the stimulus *element* in the set: for the diagnostic set, Oc (patient A) – Label of A, Oc (patient B) – Label of B, … Oc (patient N) – Label of N for the weight set, Oc (patient B) – Weight of B, Oc (patient C) – Weight of C, … Oc (patient N) – Weight of N.[24]

These relations to behavior and occasions may be depicted as in Figure 2.2.

Where control by this contingency rule (set) temporally precedes Oc-B, it is designated instructional control and typically characterizes perception research, teaching, transmission of rules. Where control by this contingency rule derives from prior Oc-(B→S) relations, it is designated abstractional control and typically characterizes abstraction concept formation research, concept awareness, induction of rules. Either way, the control is over the Oc-B relation (over Oc, B, or the relation), and such control depends upon Oc-(B→S). It should be reiterated that instructional–abstractional control is independent of awareness, ability to verbalize, etc., and is dependent on the contingencies that govern both classes of events.

One further point that is frequently overlooked will be made. Since in animal discrimination research, the subjects are typically not told the rule in advance, any rule control must emerge during the experiment. Such emergence also characterizes human abstraction and concept formation research. Accordingly, procedures that produce animal discrimination and facilitate its analysis are highly relevant for the production and analysis of human abstraction and conceptualization (cf. Goldiamond, 1962) and its distortions (Goldiamond, 1964).

Behavior analysts make programmatic plans for subject and patient behavior. Through application of appropriate controls, one can transfer such planning to one's own behavior. One then applies those requirements for self-help and for awareness relevant to self-control, which are specified by the model (Goldiamond, 1965b, 1976b). Transfer of control to the patient is a goal of most psychotherapeutic and other mental health programs.

2.5 OTHER CONSEQUENTIAL SYSTEMS

Charges of narrowness, and of the exclusion of the meaningful through rigorous application of a system, have been leveled by the nonacademic against the academic, by the literate culture against the scientific, by traditional approaches against traditional behaviorists, and by traditional behaviorists against radical behaviorists. In the present section, I shall note that the consequential approach and the logic of radical behaviorism are relatable to significant developments in social science and biological science. The developments are closely linked to each other. The interrelations are often overlooked partly because of the different language systems used, which designate identical relations in different terms, and partly because they reside in different disciplines. The questions they seek to answer, and the approaches and stances they take, relate to different significant problems that characterize the different parent disciplines. What one discipline regards as critical, another may regard as well formulated or trivial. Accordingly, well-developed formulations in one area may, if appropriately translated, obviate the necessity to develop such formulation in another. Exploring commonalities may then be of interest.

2.5.1 Cognate consequential systems in social science

Exchanges of services or commodities or both have entered into human interactions since at least the beginnings of recorded history. Indeed, among the earliest clay tablets are mercantile accounts. To condense the fine grain of interchanges between buyer and seller, I shall simply note that the behaviors of one are the occasions and consequences that bracket the behavior of the other. Thus, for the buyer, the display and ultimate delivery are stimuli that bracket buying; these stimuli derive from merchant behavior.

Merchant behavior, in turn, is bracketed by stimuli that derive from buyer behavior. In such interchange, a particular event is simultaneously the S of one and B of the other, producing parallel extended chains. Maintenance of both chains depends on reinforcement of behavior elements of each. These explicit interchanges of the marketplace are metaphorically extended to other social relations through analytic systems that then retain the terminology of the originating marketplace. Examples are *transactional* theory in anthropology and sociology and *exchange* theory to sociology, which analyze the mutual maintenance of social interchanges.[25] Their relation to the formal statements of radical behaviorism is evident upon examination of the explicit diagrams in Skinner's analysis of verbal interchange between two people (1957, Fig. 16, pp. 38, 39, 57, 84, 85). These utilize parallel lines for each speaker, in which the behavior of one is a stimulus of the other in extended chains. The different notational systems may include terms such as S^D, S^r (defined by whether the behavior of one occasions or maintains the behavior of the other), roles (defined by the nature of what one "exchanges" for what the other does), obligations (requirements for behavior). Such differences in terminology are related to differences in the parent disciplines (psychology, sociology, and anthropology, respectively). They obscure the otherwise striking similarities in the common functional analyses employed. Indeed, the sanctions of social science are functional equivalents of the aversive stimuli or negative reinforcers of behavioral psychology and of the disincentives of economics.[26]

In each of the foregoing systems of interchange, for any one of the actors, behavior may be followed by a consequence, which maintains the Oc-(B→S) relation or which strains it (if the S is a disincentive). However, in cost–benefit analysis (or benefit–cost analysis), behavior results in *two* consequences, one favorable and one unfavorable. That which is gained is accompanied by costs or penalties. In economics and planning, these are generally stateable in quantifiable terms. The relevance of the method of analysis to problems in mental health is exemplified by the psychotherapeutic adage that patients do not come in for treatment unless they are hurting, that is, the costs outweigh the benefits – as long as this relation is reversed, they will not come in for treatment. Here, differences in *explicitness* between the policy and clinical approaches have obscured the similarities in functional analyses. The extension of cost–benefit analysis to clinical problems also suggests a different interpretation of these problems. Rather than regarding the behavior of patients as pathological and irrational, we may regard it as rational – if we consider it in terms of both its costs and benefits.[27]

Rationality or, rather, the various types of rationality, are explicitly defined in decision theory. As employed in economics, the person is to choose or decide between at least two courses of action. Depending on the states of the environment, the outcomes of these actions

TABLE 2.2
2 × 2 matrix depicting the relation of courses of action and states of the environment.

Courses of action	States of the environment	
	State 1	State 2
Course 1	Outcome a	Outcome b
Course 2	Outcome c	Outcome d

will differ. For two patterns of behavior, intersecting with two possible environments, a 2 × 2 matrix is described, with a total of four outcomes entered (see Table 2.2). (There may be more than two patterns and more than two states, making for a larger matrix, but the rationale is the same, and the minimal case, of 2 × 2, will be considered here.) The environments may have different a priori probabilities, which will enter into the decision, as will the different outlays (efforts) of the different behaviors; the effects of these will be entered. (Again, for simplicity, I shall consider the a priori probabilities and outlays to be equal.) A decision criterion or *rule* must now be applied to the matrix. The rule may be to *optimize utility* (produce highest net for gains minus losses); it may be a *minimax* (gains are to be such that losses do not exceed a given [maximal] level, in one form); it may be a *maximin* (losses are tolerated provided gains do not fall below a given level in one form); it may be any of a variety of other explicitly stateable rules. The choices will be adjusted to produce those four entries in the consequence (or "payoff") matrix that satisfy the particular decision rule. This system of analysis (Von Neumann and Morgenstern, 1947) is one of the most significant advances in economics and is being extended to other disciplines in the social sciences (Luce and Raiffa, 1957), perception and psychophysics (Green and Swets, 1966; Swets, 1967; Egan, 1975), clinical decisions in radiology (Lusted, 1971), and speech classification (Karp, 1975), crime (Backer and Landes, 1974), among others. It appears to have implications for mental health as well.[28]

The system may be used in two ways, normatively and descriptively. In the normative use, the statement to a manufacturer might be, "If you are to optimize net (etc.), then you will have to take the following into account, and you *should* then follow this strategy for deciding when to buy, sell, etc."[29] In the descriptive use, one might examine (a) the long-term patterns of *behaviors* under scrutiny, (b) the various *occasions* for them, and (c) the *consequences* that occur when occasions studied and behaviors scrutinized intersect, and then (d) try to ascertain what particular decision rule or *abstractional control* is satisfied, rationalized, or specified thereby. The assumption is that the differential probabilities of the two classes of behavior ("preponderant direction of choices") are rational, that is, that *a decision rule can be specified that describes the data*. The burden of rationalization is therefore upon the investigator, and the behavior "makes sense." That this is not farfetched will find support from a different vantage point, when I discuss evolution, next. Be this as it may, this entire descriptive analysis is post hoc and suffers from the weakness of all such analyses: any of a number of after-the-fact analyses can be made. Which is then accepted may depend as much upon the ingenuity of the writer in relating it to some worldview as it does upon its fit. However, there is a way out. Given post hoc decision analysis, one can then set up an experimental situation designed in accord with it and, by manipulating variables thereby designated, predict or, more strongly, produce specified behavior.[30]

Subjective terminology is often applied in economics and other disciplines (the person *decided*, *chose*, *adopted* this strategy, etc.). However, each term so designated has an explicit referent that can be described as well without such terms. It is the functional relations between the terms and use of the terms in the explicit manner indicated that define whether the requirements of decision theory are met. If manufacturers want to know what to do and what course of action they should decide upon, the economic adviser will *translate* their terms into the explicit ones discussed. Undoubtedly, people mull over their possible courses of action and think about them. They will allocate their resources in a given way. As market conditions (or signal-noise ratios, payoff matrices, etc., in perceptual research) change, they may think differently and "chew over" something else. They may allocate their resources in a different way. Rather than state that their altered thinking altered their behavior (changed Oc→changed M→changed B), or that their altered behavior altered their thinking (changed Oc→changed B→changed M), we might state that decision thinking, planning, etc., and decision behavior both *changed as functions of the changed contingencies.*

Again, as in my discussions of emotions and awareness, it should not be assumed that both decision thinking and decision behavior follow identical relations to contingencies, no more than different classes of behavior will. And, because one can occur without the other, or one can precede the other, it should not be inferred that priority of importance or causality have been demonstrated.

The formulations of radical behaviorism are in accord with the consequential systems noted. While the problems to which it is addressed, by virtue of its narrower laboratory base, are not so encompassing, in social terms, as those of the latter, the same base has provided experimental support for the common systems and the means for such validation, which is not so readily available in the more social sciences. The complementary nature of these differences when the same system is applied to different disciplines would appear to have implications for these disciplines. At the very least, the one is not so narrow as is generally thought, and the others are not so untestable as is generally thought.

2.5.2 Biological evolution as a cognate system

To illustrate the parallelism between evolutionary theory and radical behaviorism, I shall present a thumbnail sketch of a critical problem to which evolution is addressed and the solution offered. In parenthesis next to each important evolutionary term, I shall insert a corresponding behavioral term. The reader can read the sketch twice, substituting behavioral terms for evolutionary terms, or once to note the parallelism.

2.5.2.1 *The species (behavior) problem*

Given the thousands of species (patterns of behavior) that exist, with similarities and differences between them, how does one account for these phenomena? One way, of course, is to relate them to environmental differences and similarities. If one classifies species (behavioral) environments into categories such as frigid, tropical, forest, desert, ocean (social class, culture, town size, schools attended, parental characteristics of various types, including psychological), among others, one would have to be nonobservant not to note environmental relations to species (behavior). On the other hand, one would have to be foolish to assume that speciation (behavior differentiation) is accounted for thereby, since there are obvious species (behavior pattern) differences within the same environment, hence the exaltation of correlation coefficients.

Accordingly, complex theories are developed that center around hypothesized properties assigned to species (behavior patterns of an individual) that differentiate one from the other, e.g., entelechy or species fulfillment (e.g., personality structures or dynamics). A major contribution of Darwin (Skinner) was to note that if environmental differences were treated with the same fine-grain detail accorded to species (behavior) differences

(20 feet up a tall tree in a forest might be classified as "forest environment" along with 40 feet up it [a variable 20-second *interval* schedule might be classified as an "intermittent food schedule" along with a variable *ratio* whose reinforcements were equally spaced], but these are different environments, and different species of insects [patterns of behavior] may be found), then lawful relations between environments and species (behavior) can be specified, given certain assumptions. A major assumption necessary is that offspring of a biological family (repetitions of members of a class of behavior) are not identical but differ. For a given environment, certain of the members will have a higher probability of survival (reinforcement) and, for a different environment, other members. The environment, so to speak, *selects* which members survive (remain in the repertoire) to produce further offspring (to recur); differences between these will be *selected*, and so on. Thereby, over the course of thousands of generations over time (of occurrences of behavior over a lifetime), certain biological traits (behavior classes or sets) will be established and maintained, others will be changed (shaped), others extinguished, etc. Species (behavior) stability over thousands of years (lifetime, generations) are relatable to environments that are stable with regard to those features that interact with the individuals (behaviors). The selection rule is survival–extinction (reinforcement–extinction).

Needless to say, there was more to the theory than this, as there is more today, but this suffices heuristically at this point in the discussion. Membership in groups has effects, as it does in radical behaviorism (for both social groups and groups of behavior patterns), but this discussion will be temporarily deferred. Darwin (Skinner) has been accused of not having a theory and of simply being descriptive. However, the accusation of theoretical simple-mindedness may be countered by a *tu quoque* accusation against its makers of *environmental* simple-mindedness or oversimplification. Both "descriptive" and "theoretical" positions are each complex *and* simple. One treats the environment as *complex* and thereby relates species (behavior) differences to it in a *simple* manner. The other treats the environment as *simple* and thereby relates species (behavior) differences to it in a *complex* manner.

As is evident, radical behaviorism can be considered as an application of an evolutionary model to behavior. The parallels are treated in detail by Gilbert (1970), to whom I am indebted for many of the points raised here. Typically, when application is made, it is of a natural selection of behavioral traits homologous to the natural selection of physiological traits, i.e., through genetic selection. As will be discussed shortly, an evolutionary alternative to genetic selection is possible. Be this as it may, the present discussion suggests that applications of evolutionary models to behavior can be parallel on analogous grounds (**s:e::b:e**, species are to their environments as behaviors are to their environments), as well as be homologous (s(b)°s(p) (selection of behavioral traits functions identically to selection of physiological traits).

2.5.2.2 Purposiveness and teleology

A source of the accusation against radical behaviorists that they deprive mankind of purpose should now be clear. This source is a misreading of the parallel between evolutionary theory and radical behaviorism. Since environments select *biological* traits, it is considered teleological thinking to attribute such selection to the species, i.e., giraffes developed long necks *in order* to reach the leaves of trees, rather than giraffes with long necks had a greater probability of survival in overgrazed plains. In parallel manner, it would appear to be teleological thinking to attribute *behavior* selection to the individual, i.e., the child developed (learned) a scatological vocabulary speech *in order to* win approval of peers, rather than the child's "dirty" words had a greater probability of reinforcement in the street gang. It is this audience that "selects," i.e., will reinforce scatological terms more readily than other terms.

The neck and speech analogies are exact. Presumably, arguments advancing purposiveness and thinking to explain the changing *behavior* of children should be paralleled by arguments advancing teleology and group-mind to explain the *evolution* of species. The inference follows logically and has created problems for those who, on the one hand, accept biological evolution and who, on the other hand, accept the existence of purposive behavior. There are at least four possibilities here. We should either (a) dispense with purposiveness and thinking (*p&t*) to explain the behavior of individuals (x[*b* of *i*]) and thereby avoid the embarrassment of postulating teleology and (species) mind (*t&m*) to explain the evolution of species (x[*e* of *s*]), or (b) accept (*p&t*) to x(*b* of *i*) and thereby accept the permissibility of (*t&m*) to x(*e* of *i*), or (c) accept (*p&t*) to x(*b* of *i*), but reject (*t&m*) to x(*e* of *s*) and thereby discard the effort to develop parallel psychological and biological theories, especially where humankind is concerned, or (d) accept parallelism between behavior patterns and species when behavior is not relatable to purposiveness and thinking (e.g., reflexive, automatic, instinctive), but reject parallelism when it is, that is, then accept (*p&t*) to x(*b* of *i*) and reject (*t&m*) to x(*e* of *s*); we reconcile the former parallelism [of (*b*, *i*) and (*e*, *s*)], and the latter nonparallelism [of (*b*, *i*) and (*e*, *s*)] through postulating the *emergence* of a special property of individuals when *intelligence* is evolved; purposiveness and thinking are properties of intelligence.

Each of the four positions stated is readily relatable to stances in science, literature, and philosophy. Such differences notwithstanding, they all reflect concern over parallelism between explanation of behavior change and species change. This discussion opened with an assertion that it is a misreading of radical behaviorism to equate it with depriving humankind of purposiveness and thinking. Yet, position (a) seems closest to radical behaviorism, and that position does seem to deprive humankind of purposiveness. The key is the emphasized phrase in the *use* of purposiveness and thinking *to explain the behavior* of individuals. Such use follows the linear model of causality of behavior discussed earlier, M(*p&t*)→B. As was noted in the discussions of emotion, awareness, abstraction, and decision-making, rejection of the linearly causal use of these terms does not imply the rejection of their *existence* by radical behaviorism. Rather, it implies their treatment in a different manner. If the contingencies change so that consequences available earlier for a small outlay of behavior now require a considerably higher outlay (which preempts outlays for other important consequences), the pattern of behavior may be disrupted, alternative patterns followed by other consequences may become more frequent, and so on. In such cases, one's stated goals or purposes may change before behavior changes ("I'm switching *in order to* …"), or after it changes ("Now I realize what I must have been after …"), and similar inferences may be drawn for other behavior and thinking. The same relation between *p&t* and behavior may be drawn as was drawn earlier between each of the other subjective states discussed and behavior, namely, both *p&t* and behavior *change as functions of the changed contingencies* and their histories. The functional relations need not be identical.

If one accepts certain thought patterns as abnormal, in the statistical sense, related abnormal behavior need not be interpreted as caused by the thinking, nor as the cause of the thinking, nor as yet another symptom (along with the thought "disorder") of an abnormal state. Both behavior and thinking may be relatable in an orderly manner to atypical contingencies, present or past.

2.5.2.3 *Natural selection and breeding*

Environmental change may shift survival probabilities for different members of a species, thereby changing the species over time. Changes in cellular environment may influence reproduction of genes; mutations that do not survive at one time may survive at another, when a changed environment "selects" differently. In all events, thousands of species are with us, with both similarities and dissimilarities in structure and behavior. Humans enter the scene in at least two different ways. Through predation, intrusion, and our works, we alter the environment to create new selection factors. We also function as explicit evolutionaries when we produce, through attenuation by culling and through selection for breeding, changes in species characteristics. The implications for behavior have more support than simple analogy to evolution. Before presenting such support, I shall note some precautions.

The study of past physical evolution is, theoretically, the study of past selection by previous environments. Much of this has been accomplished through tracing the history of species and by relating given structures to earlier ones. While the fossil records may present reasonable grounds for inference, the relations of the behaviors of those organisms to the fine grain of their environments are by no means so clear.[31] And it was upon fine-grain relation that the Darwinian contribution rested. Case histories in illness, whether organic or mental, often share a similar discrepancy between the comparative fine-grain of the history of the problem and the gross report of its selecting environments. Such etiologies are analogous to a descent series of fossil records: precaution is suggested.

Two other evolutionary trends suggest precautions regarding the uses to which etiology may be put in the effort to understand present behavior. These evolutionary trends are divergent and convergent evolution. In divergent evolution, variant structures may function considerably differently but may have been evolved from identical structures. The bat's wing and the human hand are, of course, ready examples of divergence from the same structure. In convergent evolution, similar structures that function similarly may have evolved from different structures. That the bat structure mentioned is called by a name ("wing") used for bird structures is a case in point. A pair of more striking examples of convergent evolution is the Tasmanian wolf and the timber wolf. Both share commonalities in appearance and behavior (hence the application of the more common name) but have markedly different ancestries, the one being a marsupial and the other a carnivore.

In divergent environmental selection of behavior patterns and thought patterns, patterns that at present differ considerably may have had common origins. Specifically, a variety of normal and, say, schizophrenic patterns may have diverged from common childhood patterns or common genetically induced patterns. One implication is that given *common*, say, genetically induced schizophrenic patterns, the outcome need not be schizophrenia. The starting patterns can be shaped to a variety of considerably different patterns. In convergent environmental selection of behavior patterns and thought patterns, patterns that at present are considerably similar may have had markedly different origins. Specifically, common schizophrenic patterns may have converged from different childhood patterns or different genetically induced patterns. One implication is that because we trace a given pattern to a certain source, then other such patterns need not derive from that source but may derive from others. Yet another implication is that, given silk and a sow's ear, we may be able to fashion equally useful purses from both.

Explicit and implicit contingency programing will now be considered. Their relation to genetic and other variables will follow, under the next topic, the origins of behaviors.

2.6 PROGRAMING AND PARADIGMS

Commenting on the demonstrated ability of radical behaviorists to train animals, that is, to change their present repertoires to explicitly specified outcome-repertoires, the authors of a textbook on learning theory noted:

> It is not wise to dismiss [these] as merely signs of cleverness on the part of the trainers. These practical demonstrations serve as important empirical supports for certain aspects of the system – a

kind of support very much needed for learning theories, and notably lacking thus far. No other learning theorist has been able to train an animal before an audience in a prompt and predictable manner … [thereby] epitomizing the principles of his theory. … [Other] demonstrations have generally relied upon exhibiting the results of earlier training. By contrast, Skinner's pigeons can be brought before a class and taught various tricks before the eyes of the audience.

(Hilgard and Bower, 1966, p. 144)

Such training involves (a) explicit specification of the *outcomes* desired, (b) selection amid all the possible *current repertoires* of an individual, of those repertoires that seem to be the most *relevant* sources of the desired outcome, (c) the explicit postulation of the series of transitional repertoires and conditions necessary to transform the present patterns into the outcomes desired, that is, the *change procedures*, and (d) the reinforcement of such transitional patterns when they occur, to *maintain* the directionality specified. These four explicitly defined elements, namely, outcome, current relevant repertoire, change procedures, and maintenance, enter into a *program*, as the term is used in radical behaviorism. As is evident from the foregoing description, behavior (among other contingency elements) is being bred. Changes in repertoire characteristics are specified, those patterns that are most promising are selected, and so on. The evolutionary model is thus not a simple metaphorical analogy. There is almost a point-for-point correspondence between the elements and relations of natural selection and of programing repertoire change. A further correspondence is that such change is accomplished through *meticulous attention to the fine grain* of the behavior, of the consequences, of the occasions, and especially of the contingency relations between them, to an extent not found in other branches of psychological laboratory research. Generalizations (laws) are based on literally tens of thousands of occurrences of behavior, recorded under one condition, then another, and so on, by a single organism run daily for as much as two hours and in some instances for over two years (see Sidman, 1960b, for the rationale).[32] Such generalizations have led to the development of a technology of programing that is related to the basic experimental analysis of behavior in the same manner that engineering as a technology is relatable to physical science.[33]

Contingency elements other than behavior may be systematically programmed and shaped. The *occasions* may be arranged and subtly changed so that children with developmental delays who were considered untestable, but who initially discriminated between light and dark (by pressing a lighted panel rather than a dark one), wound up discriminating between ellipses with an eccentricity of .95 and circles (eccentricity 1.00) (Sidman and Stoddard, 1966).[34] Such programmed change of occasions is called fading. The *consequences* that maintain behavior may be changed, so that consequences hitherto ineffective become effective – a dramatic example being the *maintenance* of behavior through providing electric shock as its payoff (Morse and Kelleher, 1970). The scheduled *contingencies* may be changed so that 75,000 responses are required to produce a consequence – and the pattern is not disrupted. Complex programs that alter combinations of these elements and their relations have also been reported (Premack, 1976); in this case, laboratory investigations of establishment of language in chimpanzees are being extended elsewhere to program such establishment for children with cognitive disabilities – an excellent example of the relation of laboratory investigation to application.

The four program elements noted are explicit in programmed instruction (*p.i.*) (Hendershot, 1967, 1973; Markle, 1975), where textbook (or other) material is explicitly programmed. The (a) outcome is given by the title of the program; (b) current relevant repertoire is given by the introduction, which states the course requirements; (c) change procedures are in the individual frames in which the student writes an answer, with the change from one frame to the next being the behavior required, or the stimulus relations to it, or both; and (d) maintenance is typically through successful progression through the program. Each frame is then a miniprogram – (a) the outcome of the preceding frame becomes (b) the current relevant repertoire for the next one. The occasions (frame material), behaviors (answers), consequences (advance to next), and contingency relations (advance when correct) of the three-term contingency are evident. It should also be apparent that changes produced by *p.i.* are not confined to the observables of the three-term contingency. Sidman and Sidman's neurology text (1967), for example, teaches the student participant *knowledge* of this field, and the first programmed text (Holland and Skinner, 1961) taught a method of *thinking* about behavior and the contingencies into which it enters. Stated otherwise, the explicit programs of radical behaviorism can change not only behavior (and the contingencies governing it) but also those private events governed by the same contingencies that govern the behavior.

2.6.1 Implications for mental health

Derived, as the system is, from the learning laboratory (although the technology extends further), the outcomes of the programs are the establishment and *construction* of new *repertoires*. The programs in *p.i.* and elsewhere are devoted not, for example, to undoing spelling errors but rather to teaching correct spelling. The program titles, which specify the outcomes, are classified by commonalities in that which is to be established (e. g., mathematics, physics, composition), as are university departments. The thrust of the programs is not to eliminate the entering ignorance, alleviate it, cure it, or teach the student to live with or adjust to it. Entering students are not assigned to classes (or programs) on the basis of their deficiencies, but rather on what they are to learn and how far they have come up to now, that is, their strengths. The contrast with conceptualization in mental *illness* is striking. I have commented elsewhere upon the distinction between the constructional or programing approach and the pathological approach that presently pervades the field:

> Help is often sought because of the distress or suffering that certain repertoires, or their absence, entail. The prevalent approach at present focuses on the alleviation or the elimination of the distress through a variety of means that can include chemotherapy, psychotherapy, or behavior therapy. I shall designate these approaches as pathologically oriented (pathos, Gr., suffering, feeling). Such approaches often consider the problem in terms of pathology which – regardless of how it was established, or developed, or is maintained – is to be eliminated. Presented with the same problem of distress and suffering, one can orient in a different direction. The focus here is on the production of desirables through means which directly increase available options or extend social repertoires, rather than indirectly doing so as a byproduct of an eliminative procedure. Such approaches are constructionally oriented; they build repertoires.

The fact that the outcomes are described differently is not simply a matter of verbal redefinition. The differences that can result become clearest when considered in terms of the four elements of a program, previously noted:

1. *Outcomes or targets.* Although similar outcomes may be produced by the two orientations when viewed in terms of distress alleviated, the outcomes of the two approaches are not necessarily similar when viewed in terms of repertoires established. For example, in a series of treatment sessions, one can progressively decrease stuttering and thereby increase the ratio of fluent words to total utterances. One can progressively instate and extend a specific fluency pattern that consists of well-junctured speech and thereby increase the ratio of fluent words to total (and decrease stuttering). Viewed in terms of

elimination of stuttering or increase in fluency (the alternate statements can simply be verbal redefinition), the outcomes may be similar. However, viewed in terms of patterns established, the outcomes may be quite different. And the training procedures and other program elements must also differ. This raises questions about outcome comparison.

2. *Current usable (relevant) repertoires.* Where the outcomes, in terms of repertoires to be established, differ, the search for what is currently relevant must be oriented differently. For example, one can focus on (and try to describe) what is wrong, or is lacking, in order to correct it. In the other case, since one is trying to construct new repertoires, one must focus on what repertoires are available, present, and effective. Accordingly, different data bases are required. Where there is overlap in the data bases, they can be interpreted differently. For instance, one can consider the presenting symptoms as among the pathologies to be overcome or eliminated; they can be considered as indicators of pathology to be specified. On the other hand, the presenting symptoms can be considered as among the entry repertoires available for construction or program guidance; they can be considered as successful instruments that produce reasonable outcomes to be specified and harnessed. For example, a pervasive cockroach phobia can be interpreted as an unreasonable fear that is so crippling to the wife that she cannot move from room to room unaided. On the other hand, it can be interpreted as highly successful instrumental behavior that dramatically forces the husband to provide the legitimate attention that he had hitherto withheld and deprived her of. The program thereby initiated is to teach him to be responsive to her legitimate needs and to teach her to express these in ways that get across to him more readily.

3. *Sequence of change procedures.* Given different target outcomes and different starting points selected for their relevance to the outcome, the mediating procedures that convert entry repertoire to target repertoire must also differ. The data that are considered as designating progress will differ, as must assessment of therapeutic effectiveness. In the phobia case just cited, although the phobia may progressively diminish, the graphs will be of increasing communication. In the case of a severely regressed person with schizophrenia, the change procedures have involved instatement of a multitude of specific repertoires, some in sequence and some concurrent.

4. *Maintaining consequences.* The contingencies of which each of the steps in a program is a component may also differ in pathologically and constructionally oriented programs. The consequences in one case may be progressive relief, diminution of aversive control, or gradual progression to such relief. In the other case, they may be explicit reinforcement of units in a progression or gradual progression toward the repertoire to be established. In the latter case, assessment concentrates on reinforcers in the natural environment. These reinforcers can be those that have hitherto been disrupting behavior. For example, a mother considers herself at a loss in rearing her son. His obnoxious behavior continually enrages her, and both his misbehavior and her rage are increasing. She reports that she is a complete failure. Our analysis is that she is a complete success. She has successfully shaped escalating misbehavior by ignoring it when it was mildly disturbing and acting only when it had exceeded the previous limit to her tolerance. This suggests that her attentiveness is a powerful reinforcer. His main way of getting it now is by infuriating her. She is to use this reinforcer to maintain progression through a different kind of program she will apply.

The symptom whose elimination is the target of a pathological approach may be considered not only as a currently usable repertoire (the cockroach phobia mentioned) but also as an important guide to critical reinforcers. For example, an obsessional patient talked rapidly and almost without stop about emanations attacking her thoughts; her eyes were piercing, and she was agitated throughout. She had been an inpatient on and off and an outpatient for 20 years. Her black and purple costume made her immediately recognizable at the emergency room, which immediately sent her to psychiatry. She was supported by a small pension and lived alone and friendless in a small rented room. In the event that she was "cured," what could she find to occupy her all day? At the present, she came to the hospital and met all kinds of different and bright people who cared. She belonged – she had community. If we were crazy enough to think we could "cure" her, she was not crazy enough to be "cured." Such elimination had been the thrust of the various preceding therapeutic efforts, which had made little progress. We told her that regardless of her behavior, she was always welcome: she was a permanent part of hospital records and was provided access to them. Community was a critical reinforcer, and the intervention strategy opened with this provision while developing other contingencies (Goldiamond, 1974, pp. 14–16).

Such programs are not confined to consulting room treatment of a single patient. For example, Keehn, a radical behaviorist of standing, set out to observe skid row alcoholics in Toronto, using such an approach, rather than accepting their alcoholism as a symptom of behavioral or mental pathology or as an effort to escape from unacceptable self or reality. Many of the alcoholics once had established professional careers that were now closed to them; they had been disowned by their families and previous referent groups. They were outcasts. There was, however, one place where they had community, and in contrast to the obsessional patient described, who found it in psychiatry, they found it on skid row. The operant behavior required for such reinforcement was buying and sharing liquor. Any ensuing medical or legal complications were the unfortunate costs attached to such behavior. The program established by Keehn and his colleagues involved providing the critical consequence of community by means of a farm leased by the provincial government. Membership in that community was open to the alcoholics, contingent upon change in their drinking patterns so that the province's costs in terms of medical and police intervention would be diminished. The members of the commune themselves set up the programs for each other, with the consultation of the staff (Keehn et al., 1973). As was noted in the introduction to a report on the program some six years after its inception,

> We assume that in the skid row inebriate there is some repertoire of behaviors appropriate to larger society. We accept the theory that new behavior can be learned and that a man's self-image can be profoundly influenced by helping him build up an investment of appropriate behaviors. We have adopted self-determination and self-help as the best means of behavioral change. We believe that a separate community is required because of the special needs of skid row people, but, although it is separate, we want it to be open to the larger community so that segregation is minimized.
>
> (Collier and Somfay, 1974. p. 6)

Fairweather et al. report a program with a similar community rationale involving considerable self-determination by long-term residents of a mental hospital. "It is possible," they conclude, "that this kind of focus on social-problem solution will turn attention once again to the creation of social systems which are fitted to human needs" (1969, p. 343).[35]

One aim of individual psychotherapy, of course, is for the patients to be able to manage their own lives. The attainment of this aim suggests to one school that treatment start off and continue to be nondirective, to others that treatment open with explicit intervention (hence the term), which is gradually withdrawn as patients improve. A radical behaviorist approach with individuals would not differ from the approach to groups suggested by Keehn et al. and

Fairweather et al., among others. This involves the development of the program in conjunction with the patient. To cite one successful outcome:

> As an illustration of how collegiality arrangements of the type discussed can lead to application of professional analysis and intervention by patients for their own problems, I shall cite the report of an outpatient upon his return from vacation. He had had a history of hospitalization for schizophrenia and his brother was recently hospitalized for the same problem. During his vacation his wife walked out on him, leaving him alone in the motel. "I found myself sitting in bed the whole morning, and staring at my rigid finger," he said. "So I asked myself: 'Now what would Dr. Goldiamond say was the reason I was doing this? He'd ask what consequences would ensue.' And I'd say: 'Hospitalization.' And he'd say: 'That's right! Just keep it up and they'll take you away.' And then he'd say: 'But what would you be getting there that you're not getting now?' And I'd say: 'I'll be taken care of.' And he'd say: 'You're on target. But is there some way you can get this consequence without going to the hospital and having another hospitalization on your record?' And then I'd think a while and say: 'Hey! My sister. She's a motherly type, and she lives a hundred miles away.'" He reported that he dragged himself together, packed, and hitch-hiked to his sister who took him in with open arms. The education occurred in the process of the analysis of several months of written records.
>
> (Goldiamond, 1976a, p. 33)

2.6.2 Implications for the paradigm

As was discussed earlier (in section 2.4.2, "Awareness and contingencies"), Weiner (1970) reported that subjects confronted with a changed contingency requirement perseverated in their previous patterns, despite the penalties now attached. However, if a specific schedule was presented, the subjects could adopt the requirements that had hitherto eluded them. Stated otherwise, to program change from A to B, C was necessary as a segment prior to B. The program sequence required was ACB, or CAB. Those subjects whose *histories* prior to B had included exposure to C could master B. Those who did not have this history could not master B, unless C was then provided. Similarly, Morse and Kelleher report that to establish shock as a reinforcer, a particular program was necessary and "such dependence on history is a general phenomenon that goes beyond situations involving electric shocks. In any situation that requires a history of reinforcement, the schedule is a fundamental determinant of behavior" (1970, p. 183). To breed organisms for certain characteristics is analogous to a program to establish certain outcomes. The characteristics or outcomes at any point in the program are products of their past breeding or outcome histories. Stated otherwise, program and history are identical: *history is a retrospective attempt to state what must have been the program, viewed prospectively*. And a program that specifies the desired progressive change only in behavior will have a hard time getting there. And a history that reports only last behaviors (behavior trends, ideological trends) will be similarly defective, as was noted in the precautions raised regarding etiology and case study. The program must include the progressive contingencies, that is, the changing relations between Oc, B, Cons, and Contingency relations. The history, if it is to be adequate, must be *a history of the contingencies* that preceded the present situation.

2.6.2.1 Relations of program history to contingencies

These relations of program and history to the contingencies may be depicted as in Figure 2.3.

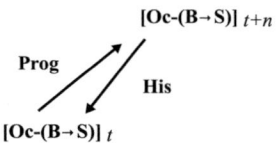

FIGURE 2.3 The relations of program and history to the contingencies

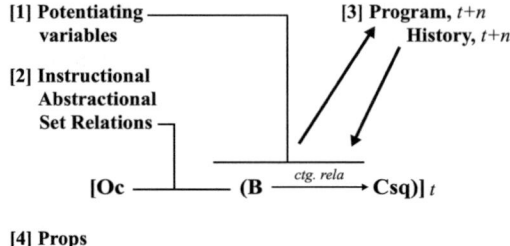

FIGURE 2.4 The simple consequential or operant paradigm

The program may be viewed as a manipulative effort to breed from a contingency at time *t* a specified new contingency at time *t* + *n*. The effort may be directed toward breeding new occasions to which behavior is responsive (fading), new behaviors (shaping), new governing consequences (change in values), or any relations of these. Regardless of which is changed, the program is effective only to the extent that all elements are considered and are effective. History is the effort to trace back a contingency at time *t* + n to earlier contingencies, *t* + *(n − 1)*, *t* + *(n − 2)*, … *t* + *(n − n)*, as far back as the historian wishes. If the historians wish to study the history of B, they must nevertheless study it in its context of bracketing occasions and selection procedures of the environment. The same would hold for trends to Oc, S, or relations between them.

It follows that whatever procedures serve to program contingencies, or to infer their histories, may also be used to program the private events represented by these contingencies or to infer their histories.

2.6.2.2 *The consequential (operant) paradigm*

As has been evident, any discussion of the three-term contingency must include more than three terms and their relations. It must include, so to speak, the supporting cast. These supports have been discussed, as in Figure 2.4, in Diagram [1], deprivational relations; Diagram [2], instructional/-abstractional set relations; Diagram [3], program history relations. One further term [4] is necessary, but its discussion can be deferred to the presentation of the combination of [1], [2], and [3] as they affect the contingency. Taken all together, they may be considered as the simple consequential or operant paradigm.

The paradigm may be depicted, in condensed form, as in Figure 2.4.

Some additional notes on these follow. For further discussion, see preceding text.

1. *Potentiating variables.* These are procedures that make the contingency potent. Deprivation of a consequence can increase its potency, and satiation refers to decrease to potency of a consequence through its presentation. Other procedures may enter (e.g., exercising, salt ingestion, or watching *Lawrence of Arabia* may increase its potency,

dietary laws may decrease potency of certain foods, etc.). The potency of behavior may be decreased by requiring too great an effort, among other means. Similarly, the potency of a schedule may be influenced by the program, among other means.

2. *Instructional, abstractional set relations.* By virtue of their close ties with the occasioning events, they follow similar relations to the contingency. They serve to select the particular stimulus (occasion) class (set), the response class (set), or both (i.e., respond to color rather than form, behave orally rather than in writing). They refer to behavior in accord with such relations, rather than to internalized understanding or abstraction.

3. *Program history.* The paradigm that is presented at any time between t and $t + n$ may be conceptualized as a slice in a progression, or as a slide in a tray of such slides. The program refers to the forward progression. The program need not be linear but can involve branching, recycling, etc.

4. *Props.* These are events that are present during the establishment, change, or maintenance of contingencies but do not enter into them. Change in the props (stimulus change) will result in a disruption of behavior, although the contingency is still in effect. Such disruption is often subjectively described as distraction, e.g., sudden noise: if the disrupting event is repeatedly or continually presented, the contingencies not having been changed, then the behavior is restored to contingency control; the props are then broadened to include such events. A program may be instituted to control for such disruption.

5. *The contingency itself.* This is presented in simplest form. The contingency may include alternative occasions, or behaviors, or consequences, or relations, either singly or in combination, as in decision theory. It may include a chain, in which each contingency is a link, as in the frames or programmed instruction (Oc_1-[B; Oc_2]-[B; Oc_3] … [B; Oc_n]). The occasions are *defined* by the contingency. Thus, the octagonal stop sign, the red light, a policeman's whistle – are all stop "signals." In the presence of any, the same [B (stop) →S (safety)] holds. Since the occasions are in the same class, any one can substitute for the others. Similarly, the behavior class is *defined* by the contingency. Stopping can involve depression of a foot brake, pulling of a hand brake, stripping the gears. The behaviors may be substituted for each other. Consequences are similarly *defined* as a class by the contingency (safety, no-ticket, stopping). Positive reinforcement is defined when (a) a consequence is presented and (b) the three-term contingency is thereby maintained thereafter. Negative reinforcement is defined when (a) the consequence consists of a *withdrawal* of an event and (b) the contingency is similarly maintained. Reversal, that is, withdrawing the positive reinforcer or presenting the negative reinforcer, may produce punishment, that is, the attenuation of behavior. In extinction, there is no contingency where there once was. Contingency relations include not only these relations but also the various schedules discussed earlier.[36]

6. *Implications of the paradigm.* If schedules are generally ignored in conventional reports of behavior, so, too, are other elements of the paradigm. In a classic study, Azrin (1958) reported that when noise was first introduced as *prop* (stimulus change), behavior was disrupted instantly but recovered under repeated presentation of noise, since the contingencies had not been changed. (Indeed, if behavior was established under noise, removing noise disrupted behavior – initially.) If, however, presentation of noise was accompanied by a schedule change that was reliably related to noise, noise served as an *occasion* for patterns of behavior specific to it. Finally, if delivery of noise was made contingent on behavior (a consequence), rate of behavior was attenuated; such delivery served as *punishment*. Stated otherwise, the effects of noise in disrupting behavior may be transient (when used as a prop change) or enduring (when used as punishment) or may be finely attuned to new patterns of behavior (when used as an occasion). Similarly, drug effects (cf. Thompson and Schuster, 1968; Weiss and Laties, 1975) are contingency-element

related. That different behaviors are tolerated under alcohol than would be otherwise suggests that it can function for the user in an instructional context: when I get stewed, different patterns will pay off. Needless to say, emotional and other states may serve similarly, in addition to serving in the various other ways suggested by an element analysis of the paradigm. And treatments that have been discarded because they have not worked may have been ineffective only because they were applied in a manner to equate them with one paradigm element. That they may be effective when used as a different paradigm element is overlooked because intervention was not analyzed in a contingency context.

NOTES

1   Skinner defines behaviorism as the philosophy of the science of human behavior and "not [as] the science of human behavior" (Skinner, 1974, p. 3).

2   There are no uniformly accepted terms. The following equivalents of reactive-consequential are to be found in the literature: (a) classical-instrumental, (b) reflex-instrumental, and (c) respondent-operant. Pairs (a) and (b) tend to be favored by traditional behaviorists and (c) by radical behaviorists, although the boundaries are permeable, and others use the terms. Earlier terms were (d) Type S–Type R, (e) Type I–Type II, and (f) Pavlovian–Skinnerian (Thorndikean). The terms reflect either history (classical, I–II. Pavlov–Skinner) or functional relation (reflex, respondent: behavior reacts to stimulus. Type S; instrumental, operant: behavior [Type R] serves as instrument or operates on the environment).

     The terms modify either conditioning, learning, response, or behavior, among other substantives. A major general textbook of experimental psychology suggests that conditioning be confined to the reactive formulation and learning or training to the consequential one, e.g., reflex, respondent, etc., conditioning and instrumental, operant, etc., learning (Kling, 1971, p. 566; cf. Goldiamond, 1975a, pp. 82–84).

3   See Leviticus 19:18; Romans 12:19; Hebrews 10:30. For further discussion of such disturbing behavior, see text.

4   In Pavlovian conditioning, a reflex (automatic S→R relation) such as blow→patellar response, and presumably innate (unconditional), can serve as a basis for a new reflex if appropriate procedures (conditions) are introduced. Thus, given (a) an unconditional reflex, US→UR (unc. stimulus, food; unc. response, salivation), if (b) a stimulus is paired with food, CS, US→UR (conditional stimulus, tone, paired with US elicits UR, since (a) US→UR still obtains, then eventually, (c) a conditional reflex will form, CS→CR (con. stimulus, tone, elicits con. response, salivation). For (c) to be maintained, occasionally (b) must also occur. Hence, the US serves to reinforce the relation. Disestablishment of a reflex through non-presentation of the reinforcer is called extinction.

5   The typical notations used by radical behaviorists are S^D-R→S^r, or S^D·R→S^r, or S^+-R→S^r. The superscripts, ^{D} and ^{r}, distinguish the two stimuli as discriminative (occasion) and reinforcing (consequences; see note 4). Both S^D and S^+ refer to presence of (B→Consequence), and S^D and S^- to absence of that relation: S^D-(B→0) or S^--(B→0). Extinction occurs under those conditions, and the organism discriminates (hence S^Δ-S^Δ) between S^Δ and S^Δ (say a red and green traffic light) by responding (stopping) differentially. I have replaced the R by a B since it is not in reaction to the antecedent, despite its historically induced persistence.

6   Thorndike formulated the Law of Effect almost 70 years ago (Thorndike, 1913). In it, as Hilgard (1948) notes, the definition of strength by probability of occurrence has "a very contemporary ring" (p. 24), with the "strengthening or weakening" a result of the consequences. Thorndike "went further and insisted that the action of consequences is direct, and need not be mediated by ideas" (p. 25).

7   Under many schedules, many instances of behavior will occur without consequences. In these situations, Oc-(B→S) relations will be observed much less frequently than Oc-(B→0). At least one psychologist has stated that when Oc-B is not followed by S, behavior is sustained by hope (for S); hope is fulfilled and sustained by the infrequent occurrence of S. If this occurs too infrequently, despair sets in, and behavior ends. (It will be noted that the mediating terms derive from the necessity of linear causality of behavior, Oc→Hope→R.) One questions the contribution of hope–despair terms when they are synonymous with the presence and absence of the observable behavior. Any procedures that influence behavior will influence hope.

     In certain forms of explanation, a particular instance is considered to be explained when it is related to a more general rule, e. g., X is jolly because X is fat follows such syllogistic format ([a] fat people are jolly, [b] X is a fat person, [c] hence …). The recurrence of B when Oc-(B→0), given only infrequent Oc-(B→S), can be explained by the schedule itself, without resort to hope. Within a very wide range, for a variety of species (rats, pigeons, monkeys), for a variety of occasions (tones, hues, patterns), for a variety of behaviors (lever-pressing, turning a wheel, making a sound), for a variety of consequences (food, water, opportunity to exercise), specifiable patterns of Oc-B (when Oc-[B→0]) will occur (behaving continually, intermittently; irregularly, regularly) depending on the (B→S) schedule (of which there are many). The schedule major premise ([a] Schedule Y behaviors are resistant to extinction, [b] Behavior X is a Schedule Y behavior, [c] hence …) has not only considerable empirical generality but also considerable experimental validation.

8   Some traditional learning theories also trivialize the status of consequences. This holds particularly for those that distinguish between learning and performance. In these models, learning is a mediating (and the crucial) concept. One can have S→L without R. In these models, for the learned behavior to occur, consequences may be necessary. Such behavior is designated as performance, and S→L→P, if C; that is, consequences are necessary for performance but not learning. Learning is inferred from changes in S→P relations for which C is necessary. In evolutionary theory, evolution does not mediate as a concept between environment and organisms. Evolution relates environment to changes in species, for which consequences are critical. See subsequent text.

9   In developmentalism, changes in behavior follow upon changes in stages of development. Physicalism is defined as a theory of knowledge that asserts that "when we introspect or have feelings we are looking at states or activities of our brains" (Skinner, 1974, p. 11).

10 Such traditional behaviorisms are designated as methodological behaviorism by Skinner (1974, pp. 13–16). This term, although regarded as "somewhat unfortunate" since it must be "distinguished from behavioral methodology" by Hayes and Barlow (1977, p. 3), is accepted by them since its use is "well-established." In Skinner's usage, methodological behaviorism is non-mentalist. However, as used in behavior modification, it is "frequently mentalistic [and] mediational," according to Hayes and Barlow. In accord with Skinner's usage, they state that methodological behaviorism is "hypothetico-deductive; relies on group designs; emphasizes pre-post measurement; and embraces inferential statistics. The philosophy underlying this paradigm is operationism/logical positivism." Those forms of behavior modification that are mentalist follow a traditional approach to linear causality. I shall juxtapose traditional behaviorism and radical behaviorism, in accord with the usage of Day (1969). He refers to conventional behaviorism in juxtaposition to radical behaviorism (p. 316).

11 The analysis of drive is a complex field, with many formulations. Their influence on disciplines outside their field varies, and my discussion centers on one particular approach that has had considerable impact outside experimental psychology, regardless of its present status within that field.

12 Both appetitive and consummatory behaviors may be considered as instrumental in obtaining consequences, but their relation to antecedents is generally linear in the drive models.

13 The physiological mediator supplies an unsatisfactory answer to the question of why food is a reinforcer. Stating that we eat because blood sugar level is down raises the question of why blood sugar is critical. If it is needed for energy, why energy? If in order to behave, why behave? If to get food, why food? And we are back to our starting point. Which discipline is propaedeutic to which depends on which arc in the circle just examined we arbitrarily study and which cut-off points we set to define the arc. By the same reasoning that we cannot understand behavior without prior understanding of the physiology of the behaving organism (see physicalism, note 9), we can reason that we cannot understand physiology without prior understanding of the psychology of the organism (cf. Skinner, 1950).

14 See note 7.

15 If only one operation defines a term, it is indistinguishable from it. (See note 7.) Cognitivist approaches distinguish themselves from mentalist approaches in that they apply converging operations to define their term and accuse mentalists of relying on only one operation.

16 For example, some time ago, S was paired with another stimulus that elicited fear and now elicits fear and anxiety on its own. Withdrawal (running), by eliminating that S, relieves anxiety, and it is this (internal) consequence that maintains the behavior. This formulation is the "two-factor" theory in which S→respondent emotion, and operant behavior has as its consequence→eliminating that emotion (see note 4). The emotion and its elimination are inferred. Other mediating formulations are used.

17 Cf. the behavior of a cornered rat.

18 We should no more expect both to be governed in exactly the same way than we so expect two different classes of observable behavior with different histories, e.g., the verbal behavior of representatives and their voting behavior. One can occur without the other. Precedence does not indicate causality: if the bear can occasion fear before I run, the bear can also occasion running before I feel frightened.

19 There is a presumption by some clinicians that what has been learned is what is actually operative; insight hence has surplus meaning beyond the congruence noted. There are other definitions of insight in psychoanalysis, just as there are in behavior analysis and in other psychologies (Goldiamond, 1977).

20 For example, in studies of concept learning with children, a series of presentations, each requiring a choice, is made. Which choice is correct has been predetermined, in accord with a concept. (The presentations may be of three triangles, in different sequences, with the middle-sized one always correct.) When degree of correctness reaches some criterion, the child may be asked to state the basis for choice, or be confronted by a different series of presentations (say, of trios of circles with a different range of sizes), or both. Which of the four possibilities discussed in the text will occur varies with experimental conditions and subjects. The definition of insight or awareness in the text intersects the one used here but is not coterminous with it.

21 Schedule A was Fixed Ratio (FR) 40 – reinforcement followed upon every 40 button presses, for ten one-hour sessions. Schedule B was Fixed Interval (FI) 10 sec. –reinforcement was delivered upon a button press occurring at least ten seconds after the last delivery; every response at some other time resulted in a loss (of 1 percent of the reinforcer). Only one button press every ten seconds was required here, but all ten one-hour sessions were characterized by the high behavior rate characteristic of FR performance. Schedule C was Differential Reinforcement of Low Rates (DRL) 20 sec. – behavior was reinforced only if the organism did not respond for 20 seconds after food delivery. Any behavior in between reset the timer to 20 seconds and delayed reinforcement by that amount.

High-rate behavior under FR is also reinforced under FI, that is, will produce reinforcement when behavior coincides with the time interval. Penultimate behavior is unnecessary but is followed by final behavior and, therefore, gain. There was a cost in the (atypical) FI schedule here. Persistence of unnecessary behavior may be related to persistence of gain. In DRL, high rate is inconsistent with any gain, hence high rate does not persist. Low-rate behavior enters the repertoire. See text for effects.

22 Cf. the army officer's maxim: "Never give an order you are not prepared to back up."

23 In perceptual research performed in accord with signal detection theory, consequences are attached to all behavior. In operant perceptual research, variable interval or ratio schedules are applied, so that behavior is occasionally reinforced. The precise relations obtained under such studies often differ from those experiments in which, once instructions are given, consequential effects are implicit, rather than explicit.

24 A form of abstractional control is contextual control. In computer terminology, instructional-abstractional control, on the one hand, and stimulus control (Oc-B), on the other, are defined as the array and the display, respectively. In a print shop, the array may be the drawers of different type fonts. The display would then be the letters in a given drawer.

25 Transactional analysis in psychotherapy has incorporated highly specialized features and internalization. In psychoanalytic theory, the explicit consequences are designated as secondary gain (because of a hypothesized primary gain). The secondary gain is stated as internalized gratification, but this is readily translatable into explicit consequences.

26 For relations to law, see Goldiamond (1976a, pp. 8–9).

27 Thus, masochism has been considered irrational and abnormal. It seems to be maintained by painful consequences that function to decrease behavior for most people rather than to reinforce it. However, masochism has rapidly been established in experimental animals. The pigeon's peck instantly delivers intense shock; the pigeon pecks again, gets shocked; continues. If no shock is produced, the bird exhibits signs of distress, moves away, may later try again, and will get back to work instantly if it shocks itself. This seems to replicate masochism, in that the organism seeks out self-induced pain. However, it turns out that when such pain is behavior-produced, so, too, is food, upon every fiftieth peck. When the shock apparatus is off, so is the food apparatus. Choice of Cost 50 shocks, Benefit one meal; Cost 0, Benefit 0, seems to be an a-rational choice, especially if the value of the meal is high because of intense deprivation (Holz and Azrin, 1961).

28 Elsewhere, I have related admission decisions to a mental hospital to such matrices, as well as relating the use of different conceptual systems to such matrices (Goldiamond, 1974, pp. 68–70). The tendency by psychiatric institutions to over-admit for suicidal threats is rational. The threatener may be admitted to the hospital or rejected. The state of the environment (person's likely behavior) may be non-suicide, or suicide. Admission of someone whose threats are idle (admit x non-suicide)→waste of money, space. Admission of someone who is serious (admit x likely suicide)→saving of life, accomplishment. Non-admission of idle threat (non-admit x non-suicide)→saving of money, space. Non-admission of someone who is serious (non-admit x suicide)→lawsuit for negligence, scandal, etc. Accordingly, the criterion for admission must be extremely low, rather than strict. Complex theories utilizing personality theory for staff have been advanced to account for what may be very simply understood phenomena (cf. Scheff, 1966, pp. 105–127).

29 Optimizing net gain is, of course, not the only possible decision criterion. When the manufacturer says: "I want to optimize net gain," he may be saying that this is what he is required to do by the stockholders. However, if an airline decides to install only that amount of safety equipment that is balanced by losses in insurance claims to the deceased, it will be in trouble. Accordingly, it may be required to apply a different criterion.

30 Control is a subset within the larger set, prediction. If one can control, one can predict. But one can predict without ability to control. Hence, both can be used for validation, but control is the stronger.

31 Since bones are calcium structures, they constitute a large part of the fossil record. However, it is the muscles that move them, and these functioning units can often only be inferred from the bones and their stress lines. And such moving units enter into behavior, which required further inference since its record is vaguest. I am indebted to Sherwood Washburn for these observations and must simply add that if behavior is inferential, the fine-grain environment contingencies are even more so.

32 In the typical psychological learning experiment, groups of organisms, separated according to experimental conditions, are run for brief periods of time. Each organism produces a small number of responses, which is entered as a single figure. Group averages of such figures are related to the conditions that distinguished them;

statistical assessment becomes necessary. The logic of the single organism and group strategies is similar, but the elements entered into the sets differ. The n (number of individuals grouped) in group research is not one in single-organism research ($n \neq 1$). Rather, n is the number of occurrences of behavior in a condition and, accordingly, n is quite large in single-organism research. The different experiments or replications run in group research are paralleled by the different individuals run under different conditions or replicated conditions.

33 The technology has entered various areas. As programmed instruction (*p.i.*), it teaches systematically what individual textbooks are designed to teach; as programmed (or personalized) system of instruction (*p.s.i.*), it is applied to systematize classroom instruction; as biofeedback, it selects for vascular, muscular, and other organic change; as behavior modification, it is extended to patterns of classroom, clinical, and industrial interest, among others; as behavioral pharmacology, it is extended to pharmacological-behavioral analysis.

34 The eccentricity of ellipse is the ratio between its minor and major axes. For a circle, the diameter is uniform throughout and, hence, the eccentricity is 1.00.

35 Braginsky, Braginsky, and Ring (1969) recommend the establishment of institutions that, in essence, provide asylum on simple request for admission, rather than making this consequence contingent on those disturbing operants that are classified as indicating mental illness. The hospital they studied had once been a private alms-house, to which the indigent reported for care. They might stay for a while, then leave. If they stayed longer, they were put to work. Many left for good; some could never get it together and returned regularly. (The poorhouse and the county (poor) farm have been abolished, of course, but there remains the problem of poverty and of people who can't get it together in the absence of programs to this end.) The investigators ran a series of studies in which patients were told that the purpose of the questionnaires was to find out who was well enough (to be discharged, in one case, or put in a privileged ward, in the other) and were told which answers indicated improvement (set *a* in one case, set *b* in the other) or deterioration. The patients presented themselves as mentally ill to stay in the hospital, or to enter it, when these served their purposes.

The poor farm origin of many of our mental hospitals is attested by the fact that in several states, such hospitals are under or allied to welfare departments (which formerly ran the farms) rather than to the health departments that regulate public health and general hospitals.

36 The following example suggests the relevance of schedules. Two pigeons are each in identical cubicles (identical props). Each pecks a disk to obtain food (Oc-[R→Csq] identical), having been equally deprived (potentiation identical). Intervals between delivery of food are, on the average, about 30 seconds apart for each. Despite all these identities in the environment, the pigeons behave differently, and when extinction is introduced (by turning off the feeder), the course of behavior will differ.

One pigeon was on a Variable Interval 32-second schedule, that is, once food is delivered, a timer withdraws the food magazine for that time interval (on the average), and only a peck after the timer has timed down and locked will deliver food. The timer will then recycle. The other pigeon was on a Variable Ratio 64 schedule, that is, once food is delivered, a counter withdraws the food magazine until that number of pecks has been cumulated (on the average), at which point, food is delivered. The counter then resets. In one case, delivery of food is contingent on a peck after a time interval (during which pecking was immaterial); in the other case, it is contingent on a peck after a given number of pecks (for which behavior is essential). The time intervals are the same, because the second pigeon pecks at a rate of about 2 per second. It is precisely such schedule relations that are critical in the world around us (piece work, pay on time, time-dictated deadlines, performance-based contracts; take every two hours, take when pain occurs, etc.) and that constitute the laboratory study of schedules that tend to be ignored when environments are typically considered, and especially so in heritability studies.

3

The origins of behavior patterns

If we question the application of linear causality to consequential behavior, that is, to behavior that is not inconsequential or trivial, what are the origins of behavior? The question is not a trivial one, nor is it paralleled by issues surrounding the Origin of Life. Genetic theories are being advanced to areas of behavior as disparate as criminality, intelligence, and schizophrenia. Physiological induction of emotional behavior has been demonstrated for some time. These propositions have not only interventive effects (genetic counseling, eugenic sterilization, chemotherapy) and social effects in terms of delivery systems and types of recipients but also effects on research and understanding. Yet another implication is the relation of behavior to evolution. If there is selection of behavior in the sense of the terms as used in biological evolution, it would appear that genetic and physiological induction are critical.

This discussion of the origins of behavior patterns will be divided into three sections. First, I shall consider some sources and relate them to environmental contingencies. Second, I shall extend the evolutionary analogy raised earlier (species change and behavior pattern change) to social inheritance as alternative for or supplement to biological inheritance of behavior, in the context of contingencies as they relate to mental health. Third, I shall consider some specific problems in mental health.

3.1 SOURCES

The major sources of current repertoires include the following.

3.1.1 Programing sources

In the same sense that certain present breeds of domesticated cattle have their origins in cattle from which they were bred, a vast array of patterns of behavior (and other contingency elements as they relate to behavior) have origins in program histories. The program may have been explicit and highly systematic, as in *p.i.*, or explicit and less systematic as in school education, or implicit, as in parental and peer requirements and interactions.

3.1.2 Reflexive sources

Certain reflexes may be capitalized upon as sources for contingency programing or reactive conditioning. The physiological apparatus of children permits vocalizations, and a *wa:wa:*

DOI: 10.4324/9781003260103-3

sound may, in certain audiences, be shaped to *wa:ta:*, in others to *vo:da*, and in yet others to *a:wa:* and so on. Reflexive swimming occurs during the first year of life and recurs in about two years. If a program is not applied, as it is in the vocalization case cited, the sources of later swimming will be in the first category.

3.1.3 Physiologically induced sources

Electrical stimulation of or surgery in certain areas of the brain can serve to reinforce preceding behavior or suppress or induce behavior: it can induce components of sexual behavior and of aggressive behavior, among others. (For an excellent review, see Valenstein, 1973.) Since there has been extensive laboratory investigation of aggressive behavior, and since it will be discussed in other contexts as well, I shall focus on this behavior. Delgado (1969, p. 129) electrically stimulated, through telemetry, the appropriate brain area of an adult female monkey. She then attacked other monkeys, S→R. However, such attack was induced by brain stimulation when she was with one group of monkeys. Stimulated similarly when in a different group, she hardly attacked. S°|R. I shall return to this later.

3.1.4 Genetic induction

The occasions available for sighted organisms differ from those available for blind organisms, and an environment with reflected light may select for one and not the other. Similarly, one would expect selection of behavior, of relation of behavior to consequences, and of other elements in the paradigm. Reflexes, susceptibility to electrical stimulation, and schedule induction, to be discussed later, also enter. The extent to which highly complex patterns of behavior are so determined is not as readily apparent but has recently been reopened in sociobiology (Wilson, 1975), in addition to its more familiar postulations in criminology, mental illness, mental testing, and linguistics. Indeed, inherited linguistic structure has now been extended to inherited ethical structures in humans to account for ethical universals (Stent, 1976).

3.1.5 Schedule-induced behavior

A variety of behaviors of clinical relevance (e.g., pica, polydipsia [Falk, 1961], defecation [Rayfield, Segal, and Goldiamond, 1978]) have been reliably induced when reinforcement has been made contingent on workaday behavior (e.g., lever-pressing for food) under specified conditions. Similarly, behaviors of social relevance have been reliably induced. Instantaneous and simultaneous attack upon each other can thereby be induced in animals who have never been together. The effects have been obtained in practically all vertebrates tested (including turtles, pigeons, rats, rabbits, monkeys). The attack conditions may be summarized as follows: (a) noxious stimulation (e.g., shock, pinch) presented freely or made contingent on workaday behavior: the stimulated animal will attack another, if present (Ulrich and Azrin, 1962), or inanimate objects, if not (Azrin, Hutchinson, and Saliery, 1964); or (b) a less favorable change in the reinforcement schedule, either through decreasing the amount or frequency of reinforcement, or increasing the work requirement for the same reinforcement, or stretching both to the limit, as in extinction, when reinforcement is absent no matter how great the effort (Azrin, Hutchinson, and Hake, 1966). If an attack object is made available only through specific behavior, an aggression-induced animal will engage in that behavior, produce the object, and attack. The opportunity to aggress thereby becomes a reinforcer for the behavior specified (Azrin, Hutchinson, and McLaughlin, 1965). The size of the enclosure is critical: if small, attack is induced; if large, escape (for comprehensive reviews, see Gilbert and Keehn, 1972; Keehn, 1976; Hutchinson, 1977; Staddon, 1977). Aggression by rats in a small enclosure may be replaced by sexual mounting in a larger enclosure upon females and males (Caggiula, 1972) and also upon inanimate objects (Caggiula and Eibergen, 1969). It can be argued that what makes aggression reinforcing similarly affects such sexual assault.

3.1.6 Relations to contingencies

The extent to which the patterns or, more precisely, their constituent subpatterns are to be assigned to one or more of the other sources noted (programing, reflexive, physiologically induced, genetically induced), or should be classified separately (schedule-induced), may depend on further experimental analysis. Regardless of source, analysis thus far suggests interesting subsequent relations to the programing environment. Given the necessary conditions for aggression for two animals, a skirmish will ensue. If skirmishes are induced on subsequent days, a change may occur within a short period of time. When the aggression-inducing conditions are now introduced, one of the animals will move to the attack. However, the other will attempt to escape or will be propitiatory. What happened was that during the skirmishes, one animal tended to win. Attack by the loser was increasingly punished. The alternative behaviors in escape and avoidance were then selected on the *occasion* of the inducing schedule change. Presumably, the accompanying emotional state was also reversed – for *one*.

We may now return to our discussion of Delgado's data in which physiologically induced aggression in one group was replaced by other behavior when electrical stimulation was then applied. The monkey had occupied a dominant social position in the one group and a subordinate one in the other. The operant contingencies supplied by the social groups swamped any physiological induction in this case (Delgado refers to such social effects as settings for the behavior). In the case of the pigeons, the development of such social contingency relations over time *reversed* the nature of the scheduled-induced behavior in one case and strengthened it in the other. Environmental contingencies also entered into the establishment or nonestablishment of reflex-based behaviors, or in the directionality of yet others, some of which are genetically characteristic of a species.

A conclusion seems inescapable. *Regardless of the source of the behavior pattern*, if the behavior affects the environment around it, once the behavior occurs and recurs, it enters the public domain, that is, the domain of its environment. And once it does so, *the source and type of behavior can be swamped by those patterns required by the consequential contingencies.*

Certain genetically induced physiological patterns may be triggered at different times by developmentally related changes. However, what public behavior is induced will be governed by not only the contingencies then extant but also the history of other members of its behavior class, during exposure to a history of past contingencies.

Indeed, humans set up social systems that maintain environments within certain ranges. Such limitations upon possible contingencies and programs will now be considered.

3.2 CULTURAL INHERITANCE

The analogy between breeding for specified traits and programing for special skills, as noted earlier, is considerably more than a metaphor. For each point in one, there seems to be a corresponding point in the other. Similarly, there is a strong correspondence parallel between natural selection applied to species and environmental selection applied to patterns of behavior.

Social and cultural systems restrict the range of contingencies, as evidenced by the fact that this discussion is being written in a language pattern into which the initial patterns of numerous other people have also been programed. The programing includes both implicit and explicit contingencies that, when applied, govern behavior with varying degrees of systematization. Such *programing behaviors* (as opposed to *programed* behavior) will have been shaped in the training and other social interaction patterns of numerous members of our culture. In certain subcultures, the contingencies governing programing behaviors will be quite similar, in others less so.

Children are trained by their parents, that is, specific parental contingencies bracket specific behaviors of their children, in a sequence that includes implicit and explicit elements. I shall assume that to the extent that the larger cultural and other environments remain consistent over time, as they have in many traditional cultures, the similar cultural milieu will maintain the applications of these training programs over generations. The programs applied by parents to their children's behaviors will be the programs applied by these children to *their* children's behaviors, when they are parents, and these children will apply the programs when they are parents, to the program-relevant behaviors of their children, and so on. I believe that it is in this context that we can speak of cultural or social inheritance (cf. Medawar, 1977), that is, the transmission of *programing procedures* from one generation to the next. (Social institutions such as schools, religious and legal systems, and professions also transmit programing procedures. These may be analyzed similarly.) Such procedures include the implicit or explicit selections of outcomes (expectations), procedures, and other program and contingency elements discussed earlier. Programing survives, like individuals and species, through environmental selection: the children do not walk off the edges of mesas and survive to transmit the programing procedures to other generations. New environments impose new requirements, and programs may change. Some changes will be in terms of a natural drift; others may be sudden and so large as to be incongruous with other critical programs maintained by the system. Yet others may be sudden but small enough to be so congruent; under certain conditions these may be perpetuated, under others not. The parallels to biological transmission, natural selection, genetic drift, mutations may be extended. We might speak of the (culturally) selfish program or the (culturally) altruistic program, as glibly as we do of such genes, or of behaviors that are only the program's way of perpetuating programs or of programs that are only the behavior's way of perpetuating behaviors.

Into this well-ordered scheme there enters an exceptional child. The child may be slow. The child's patterns of behavior or of receptivity to the environmental occasions or consequences may deviate in other ways from those typical initial repertoires to which the culturally inherited patterns of programing are geared. Such deviation can arise through amniotic poisoning or through fetal abuse by alcoholic, addicted, or psychotic (among others) mothers and fathers. It can arise through illness, accident, or related trauma. It can be *genetically induced* through transmission or mutation. Regardless of the origins, the child is either not responsive to the program or responds in ways to which the culturally inherited program is not geared. I shall note three possibilities. Others exist.

3.2.1 Parental persistence with standard programs

The parents may persist in their use of the standard program. Through failing to obtain the appropriate steps, or through being required to behave excessively to obtain these, they may exhibit schedule-induced anger or other emotional patterns. Such emotion, and the concern involved, may then become parent outcomes that shape children's patterns. It is the child's disturbing behavior that produces and may be maintained by such concern, especially if normative patterns do not produce concern so readily. And the parents, in more than one scenario I have observed, notice that they become intensely involved as a consequence of disturbing behavior and less involved as a consequence of normal behavior and, reasoning that they are "rewarding misbehavior," try to ignore this pattern. The child then escalates this pattern, with induced emotion, to the point where the parents yield. An escalated pattern has been reinforced. Over time and through repetitions, the disturbing patterns can become, within their outcome-governed limitations (control of parents), *as sophisticated and adroit as the more typical patterns are in other children.* In the meantime, the parents are so delighted over any nondisturbing behavior that they "reward it" immediately, thereby keeping it at a primitive stage in the program. In the more typical program applications, it is precisely these behaviors whose escalation and refinement the social environment progressively requires during development.[1] (Similarly, in high ratio performance, the investigator requires increasing escalation of behavior.) The solution here is to train the parents to reverse their programing procedures: yield instantly when disturbing behavior occurs, set the occasions and programs for nondisturbing behavior, and gradually escalate the requirements here. Such reversal requires considerable programing sophistication. For one thing, the child is highly adept in programing skills; for another, the parents are now required to change their patterns and develop new ones. Other problems enter.

3.2.2 Culturally available alternatives

Parents may apply alternative programs systematically available in the cultural repertoire when the standard programs do not work (see Table 3.1). The data suggest that such alternative programs are neither random nor unlimited. There may also be cultural and biological limitations.

These programs, not having been developed for all individually egregious behaviors, may result in child outcomes that, while not normative, are clustered in similar groupings, depending on the similarities between alternative programs – children repertoires.

3.2.3 Novel programing for standard outcomes

Here, the parents may implicitly or explicitly define the necessary outcomes. They may similarly select from the repertoire of the child those patterns that can be used as a basis for a program directed toward the outcomes. They may then patiently *innovate* change procedures by steps that transform current repertoires to outcomes and may apply appropriate reinforcement all along. Stated otherwise, when confronted with initial patterns that deviate from those with which culturally inherited programs and alternatives mesh, they do not attempt to apply standard programs or "compensatory" alternatives (cf. Jensen, 1969). They apply a new program based upon careful observation and monitoring of their child's behaviors, as they change theirs. Stated otherwise, they are applying, implicitly perhaps, the programing

TABLE 3.1

Possible outcomes obtained for disturbing and alternative patterns on different occasions given different programs.

Behavior patterns	Occasion 1	Occasion 2
Disturbing patterns	Outcome a	Outcome c
Alternative patterns	Outcome b	Outcome d

procedures that are explicitly defined in *p.i.* Professionals might learn from such parents. Needless to say, novel programs can also produce outcomes different from those intended.

I believe that such cultural programing inheritance accounts for the transmission of mental illness from parents to offspring, and its nontransmission – at least as well as gene-programed psychosis. One report (Heston, 1966) is of infants removed from schizophrenic mothers at birth and reared elsewhere. Follow-up when the infants were adults revealed an unusual proportion of schizophrenic and other disturbing patterns. There were also normal patterns. A genetic interpretation has been offered to counter the "schizophrenogenic parent syndrome" that has been offered as an explanation. If we assume that the neonates of the schizophrenic mothers tended to behave initially in manners to which the culturally inherited programs are not keyed, then the adoptive parents may have engaged in any of the three programing patterns noted (or others). The results obtained are as consistent with this interpretation as they are with a genetic one.

Reports of fairly uniform proportions of schizophrenia throughout the world have been interpreted to support a genetic explanation, since, after all, human beings share a common gene pool that characterizes their humanity, defined biologically. However, they also share commonalities in behavioral and other cultural patterns that distinguish them from other species. Such patterns, including the employment of language, undoubtedly aid in the cultural and social transmission of programing behaviors from generation to generation. The reportedly similar proportions of schizophrenia throughout the world may be relatable to similar proportions of different programing options and alternatives throughout the world.

Similarly, the linguistic data accounted for by inherited structures may be equally well accounted for by divergent evolution of language programing from one common source. Just as the vast majority of humans biologically descended from one source share common organs, so, too, the vast majority of language-programing procedures culturally descended from one source may share common patterns. A biological theory of evolution does not appear to be necessary to account for (genetically) inherited structure in language, or ethics, for that matter. A biological theory of evolution does not appear to be necessary to account for the replacement of one language over another, namely, that the speakers of one language had a survival edge over the speakers of another, *by virtue of* the language differences. Language programing behavior is one of a complex of social influences, which include different technologies, social organizations – and accidents of geography and history. Such accidents are found in biological evolution as well. The island on which a truly admirable species is found may suddenly sink under the ocean – through no "inferiority" of that species. And neither are survival, nor spread of language, nor ethical system, nor other programs indicators of survival value of these systems. Survival and spread may adhere to accident, to possession of best bomb, or to immunity to virulent disease.

3.3 PROGRAMING DISTURBING AND UNDISTURBING CONTINGENCIES

The proliferation of areas to which explicit programing behaviors are being applied indicates the general applicability of the consequential framework discussed, as well as supporting the relevance to behavior of a *parallel* to evolutionary selection (rather than of a homology of evolutionary selection of behavior). It would appear that there exists considerable understanding of programing procedures and contingency relations. Although these are being applied in increasing manner as a technology that can help solve behavior problems, they are unfortunately not being applied to the same extent to the *understanding* of such problems and their development.

3.3.1 Problems to understanding

In part, inattention to understanding derives from the necessity of careful monitoring of the implicit or accidental *programs* that produce such outcomes. In effect, this requires a history of not simply the behavior patterns but also the progression of contingencies, that is, the behaviors and their bracketing environmental contingencies. Such studies as have been done have been highly suggestive.

For example, Moss observed neonates at three weeks and three months and noted that even at these early ages, mothers were differentially responsive to boys and girls: they stressed musculature in boys and aroused them more; imitated their daughters more (1967, p. 27); and "in keeping with cultural expectations the mother is initiating a pattern that contributes to males being more aggressive or assertive, and less responsive to socialization" (p. 30). In another study (Moss and Robson, 1968), fretting girls were talked to and boys held (cf. Korner, 1974). In the absence of such environmental selection data, explanatory roles are assigned to inner instinctive differences (entelechies in evolution) and to terms such as attachment, but "the shortcoming of the theory of attachment … is that it does not speak sufficiently to the social interaction that is the key to socialization. Proximity is necessary but not sufficient" (Bell, 1974, p. 9). Stated otherwise, attachment omits, at the very least, the schedule.

With regard to mental illness, the problem of such observation is compounded by a selection problem. The patient whose behaviors are disturbing occasions professional attention only *after* the episodes have occurred. History must then replace direct observation of programing. While observation and programing thereafter can occur and can be used to infer previous program history, they are limited by their post hoc nature. However, it should be noted that Darwin's model did not derive from the monitoring of ongoing evolution.[2] It did, however, replace other models that internalized evolutionary processes within the species. A considerable body of *observations* buttressed the arguments advanced. While there have been some evolutionary laboratories, the behavior analysts have been in a better position. They (the environments) can change behavior patterns (species) within the laboratory by culling and reinforcing selected constituent behaviors (individuals) and can do so for extended periods of time. Of the various learning analysts, it is the radical behaviorists who are closest to this model, as Hilgard and Bowers have noted. Accordingly, there are probably many more supported relations available in this area than there were for Darwin in his time. However, several precautions should be noted.

Darwin observed and related biological phenomena *to their environments*; those behavioral phenomena which have been related to the fine-grain of their environments have generally not been the phenomena of mental health and mental illness but have involved basic laboratory behaviors. And behavioral theories in mental health have not been so encompassing as those of Darwin (for early efforts see Sidman, 1960a, 1960b; Skinner, 1956). A counterargument is that the laws of mechanics do not have to be reformulated for every different type of machine, nor should they have to be reformulated for a behavior contingency analysis of *mental* health/illness. If the scientific analogy supports the extension of laboratory behavior analysis to nonlaboratory behavior, a similar technology analogy suggests difficulties. Although the same laws of mechanics apply to both airplane and automobile motors, one would prefer an aircraft mechanic to an automobile mechanic to work with airplane motors. The automobile mechanic might replace a required light aluminum alloy part by an equally well-fitting heavy steel part. Similarly, while reinforcement principles might overlap in the school and the clinic, a school behaviorist might apply procedures in the clinic that create other problems. Accordingly, one might extend what one can and cannot apply in other science/technology relations to what one can and cannot apply in behavior analysis-application relations.

Another extension may be noted. To the extent that mental health/illness is a social problem, as well as an individual one, analysis in terms of only one area may not serve to explain the data, nor will treatment so derived. (Analogies will be found in other sciences.) Consider, for example, a hospitalized patient, in whose case magnitude of settlement of a claim will be contingent on magnitude of disability. Such outcomes can be (but are not always) highly potent. The likelihood of patient participation in therapeutic programs is remote, whether the programs involve physical therapy, psychotherapy, applied behavior analysis, behavior therapy, or any other medically sponsored treatments, including medicine itself. Typically, the patient is then classified as refractory or resistant (which are merely synonymous with what is already observed), or as exhibiting denial (which integrates the behavior with a theory assigning internal causation), or as being a goof-off or a sociopath (a characterological assignation [assassination?]). The professionals may flagellate themselves or their fields: *they* don't *know* how (internal causation), or the state of the art is not that advanced. What is at work is the social system and the resolutions of conflicting and supporting interests expressed in the laws and regulations. As Valenstein (1973) noted with regard to a related issue, "there is a great danger in accepting the delusion that biological solutions are available for these social problems" (p. 353). For biological, substitute any other solution based on individual change. With regard to behavior analysis, a consequential-contingency analysis is being affirmed, rather than denied. What is at issue is the environmental *source* of the elements bracketing behavior. In the case cited, it is under the control of the larger social system rather than of the therapist, the hospital, the family, or other subcultures. And to the extent that the societal consequences are contingent on the patient's behavior, whether or not they are delivered is under the patient's control. And that is the problem – to the "helping" professional.

With regard to present understanding, the theories that are now considered "classic" have been developed within the life-spans of most readers of this chapter. Their relationship to effective practice may be attested by the continual proliferation of new theories and treatments. Such proliferation suggests both that there is enough promise (success) in present approaches to justify the quest and that such performance is wanting in many respects. What seems to be needed is more fine-grain data, of not only the behavior patterns but also the bracketing environmental contingencies. Such data may provide not only for conceptualization but also bases for breeding new behavior patterns.

3.3.2 Some contingencies of disturbing behavior

Disturbing behavior may be viewed as behavior that disturbs others. A *unilinear* (but not necessarily linearly causal) contingency analysis might be applied to its contingencies in the following manner: for the pattern to continue, the behavior of others upon such occasion may serve as reinforcement. The likelihood of the disturbing behavior is thereby maintained or increased in the future, when the appropriate occasion occurs. Reinforcement may be negative or positive: the disturbing behavior either produces the "desired" effect or eliminates an "undesired" state of affairs. That one should want to disturb others raises questions about the pathology of the relation or of either or both of the parties. Reference is then made to the costs as well as the benefits for the person, the significant other, or both, and it is inferred that treatment will be sought only when the patient is "hurting" – that is, the costs considerably outweigh the benefits. And then, of course, therapeutic wisdom has it that the patients come to get rid of the hurt but not necessarily to change their behaviors or personalities. While the contingencies reflected undoubtedly do occasionally occur, there are more subtle and complex situations they do not describe. An analysis in terms of *alternative* contingencies, rather than unilinear contingencies (Goldiamond, 1975a), may describe both the complex situations and the (relatively) simpler ones noted. Such an analysis, of course, may be conveniently rationalized by decision theory, as well as raise programing questions.

The matrix would involve *at least* two patterns of behavior. One of these is the disturbing pattern. The other is an alternative one. (There may be other alternatives, but the analysis is not thereby complicated, although the computation may be.) If these alternatives are arbitrarily represented by rows, the occasions are represented by at least two columns. And the four cells formed by the intersections represent the consequences for the four contingencies described. Which behavior occurs will then become a function of the *resolution of the matrix* through some decision criterion, an abstractional control applied to the matrix. The explanation or the occurrence of the disturbing behavior then resides not in the "desired" effects it produces or the "undesired" state of affairs it eliminates but rather in the relation of its various outcomes to the various outcomes of its various alternatives. Adequate explanation in unilinear terms is a special case of the foregoing. It obtains when the entries in the row of alternative behavior are minor, in comparison to those in the row of the disturbing behavior. The therapist's task in psychotherapy (or behavior therapy or applied behavior analysis) may be conceptualized as reversing the direction of this difference. In those therapies using a constructional approach, the major thrust will be to raise the values of the alternatives. In constructional behavior analysis, explicit programs will be developed in this context, with outcomes specified, etc. This will especially hold where nondisturbing alternatives that stand a chance of competitive selection are almost nonexistent. Prior efforts may have been overwhelmed by environmental selection of the disturbing patterns or may not have been programed further (as was noted for the child whose disturbing skills were advanced but nondisturbing primitive) or may have been extinguished, etc. Where such alternatives hardly exist, they must first be developed before a matrix can be defined.[3] This may account for the receptivity to operant investigators by institutions for people with cognitive disabilities or for other populations where alternatives may not have been developed. Such populations should be distinguished from those that have such repertoires but whose matrix resolution overwhelmingly favors the disturbing behaviors to such an extent that the alternative repertoires seem to be nonexistent.

One further variable, relatable to the matrix, should be considered. This is the comparative behavior effort to engage in disturbing and nondisturbing alternatives. If the two levers require different force (but produce similar outcomes), choice will be affected. If the effort to shift from the present disturbing behavior to a desired alternative is greater than the net gain (or other decision criterion) described by the matrix, there may be little shift. The small steps of explicit programs reduce such effort but not necessarily the time. And if such use of time preempts the time for disturbing patterns, the benefits of these patterns are then lost. Competing benefits must then be built explicitly into program participation.[4] Another resort that finds use is to remove the individual from the environment that selectively reinforces disturbing patterns. Such removal and change of scene *in and of itself* may not be effective, unless the new environment does not so select and also selects for the alternatives in a systematic manner. Unless the comparative effort, or shift-effort, variable is considered, there may be little change. In our investigation of the contingencies governing drug addiction and its alternatives, we noted that the present patterns of some addicts had little to offer *in comparison* to the alternatives considered desirable by both the addicts and the clinics in which they were enrolled. However, in one case, developing the new repertoire would take at least two years of concentrated effort, during which time benefits of the present pattern would be absent. The present repertoire required little new effort: the addict was already engaged in it. (Although such effort, investment, cost, etc., is handled in various ways in economics, it requires special enough consideration here to require a third column in the matrix.)

In the next few paragraphs, I shall present a few patterns of disturbing behavior that exemplify the foregoing analysis. A more extensive analysis could be made, and a typology of disturbing behavior contingencies would also be more extensive. Accordingly, the examples presented are illustrative rather than exhaustive.

3.3.2.1 Social matrices

It has been noted that during economic depressions, rates of mental illness and crime may increase. These are often attributed to the personality disorganization caused by the social stress. However, army enlistments also rise. This pattern of behavior is clearly not involuntary. Examination of behavior alternatives and their consequences may be helpful. One means of obtaining necessities is through gainful employment. However, the alternative ways of doing so are limited for the urban and rural poor, and even these means are diminished during economic depressions. Alternative means of obtaining necessities are through psychotic behavior (mental hospitalization), criminal behavior (money or prison incarceration, or both), or enlistment (military). These should increase during depression.

Indeed, the clientele of mental hospitals and prisons has been drawn from the urban and rural poor, and these populations have contributed heavily to the ranks of raw recruits in the military. Which requisite behavior is "selected" will depend on the selection patterns and programs of the environments ("opportunities"). Indeed, one recidivist in a mental hospital was quite explicit when he ran through his resources; he said, he could hold up someone, "but they're as poor as I am." So, he attacked city property – in full view of two Chicago policemen; the computer printout at the station reported a psychiatric record, and he was reconsigned to the mental hospital. This patient could define the contingencies. Others may not. As was discussed earlier, whether or not the person is aware of the contingencies is irrelevant to their control. With regard to the rational–irrational dimension, appropriate payoff matrices can be assigned to enlistment in any of the institutions mentioned. In this context, the behaviors are rational. Indeed, the assignment of involuntariness and irrationality to psychotic behavior has created a difficult legal situation in the area of criminal insanity, where killers have been judged not guilty and released to kill again.

For some patients in mental hospitals, environmental programing has never been applied in a variety of life skills other than the vocational. Such programing absence is not confined to hospital populations, of course. Backwoods people have not been programed for certain living skills in a crowded urban slum – just as urban dwellers have not been programed for woods skills, and just as rural teenagers are not "street-wise." Given such urban-skill deficiencies, when mental hospitals are closed down and the formerly "warehoused" patients are consigned to retail outlets ("halfway-houses," "group homes") that are concentrated in one locality (e.g., Uptown in Chicago), they become easy prey for those elements of our urban system for whom the behavior effort–cost–benefits of predation outweigh the effort–cost–benefits attached to alternative patterns. The locality deteriorates further.

The campuses of mental hospitals could serve as programing centers for living skills, just as the campuses of other institutions program academic and vocational skills. Such skills in the latter institutions are programed for postgraduate living outside the institutions and are constructional: they classify according to the different skills to be learned, rather than attempting to cure an amorphous ignorance; they assess entering skills rather than entering deficits; and in *p.i.* and *p.s.i.* (personalized systems of instruction), they program step by step and do maintain progression with little drop out. The campuses of mental hospitals could also be so used (cf. Fairweather, 1969; O'Brien and Azrin, 1973). Instead, they are being dismantled. The societal matrices involved in such catchwords as "mainstreaming," "institutionalization," and "warehousing" are another story. In defense of Madison Avenue, "pinpoint carbonation" was never elevated to the status of the social good, true, or beautiful.

3.3.2.2 Individual matrices

The obsessional patient mentioned earlier (section 2.6.1) could either talk compulsively or speak sensibly; the alcoholics in the Keehn et al. project (same section) could drink to excess or moderately, or could abstain. However, among the benefits of the disturbing behavior for both was community membership (the costs differed for each). Among the costs of alternative behavior for both was isolation (the benefits differed). Obsession and alcoholism were rational. Such matrices are peculiar to the individuals involved and are not necessarily specific to a social class, as were the matrices of the urban and rural poor noted in the preceding section.

In both cases, programing involved making the same critical consequence contingent on alternative behaviors that lacked the high costs attached to the disturbing patterns. The alternatives were programed gradually through environmental changes planned in my office in one case, and through a separate community in the other.

3.3.2.3 Matrices involving metaphors

Phobias often enter into this category, with the cockroach-phobia patient (section 2.6.1) for example. She was immobilized thereby and her husband swept and cleaned the house every morning (to clear it of vermin), brought her breakfast in bed, and washed the dishes (to deter vermin) before leaving for work. Whenever she recovered somewhat, his attentiveness waned. The phobia was costly: she could not resume the professional work she had enjoyed, nor could they go out together at night; further, her in-laws were suggesting divorce. The benefits to recovery are obvious, as is the matrix. There is a metaphor involved. Labeling the disturbing behavior as a psychiatric problem is *essential to the matrix*. The patient would not get the accruing benefits if she simply told her husband: "Look, you've been putting work ahead of me and everything else since we've been married. I've worked to keep this marriage together. How about you?" Indeed, earlier efforts in this direction had been extinguished. *Numerous psychiatric problems have this legitimate labeling function.* Labeling theorists who denounce such terms might reflect further on this metaphorical use for the patient, rather than upon the psychiatrist's benefits and the crippling effects of the label upon the patient. *It is the contingency matrix that produces the disturbing effects* and governs the behavior *and* the experienced emotions or thought patterns.

Programing in the phobia case involved making the same critical consequence (marital involvement) contingent on alternative patterns. He was to supply this consequence and was therefore as essential to the program as his wife.

3.3.2.4 The preempted deficit

A child is attentive to her parents and other adults. Their responsivity reinforces and refines this behavior; she seeks out adults, and this successful pattern preempts interacting with peers. The deficit produced thereby may put her at a social disadvantage later. Such deficits do not seem to fit into present contingency-matrices. However, they are the programed outcomes of historically past matrix resolutions. Students who become skilled in copying from others may get good grades, but the deficit in course material may put them at a disadvantage later.

Programing involves starting with the present repertoire. She is to observe what her peers do and try to transfer some of her skills with adults to them. Programing at this late date is usually more costly than programing would have been at the appropriate time in the past (especially for the student who cheated). Now it has to be supplied; then it was available. Now the effort may compete with other benefits that were then unavailable, and an alternative contingency matrix must be considered.

3.3.2.5 *Mutual disturbance*

Parents often punish disturbing behavior, which then stops. Thereby the *child* negatively reinforces punitiveness by parents, that is, their punitive behavior (a) eliminates a state of affairs and (b) is maintained thereby: they complain that they are constantly nagging. The *parents* leave the child to his own devices when his behavior is not disturbing but are involved when it is. Parent and child mutually select for mutually distressing patterns, in a reversal of the positive interpersonal equivalent of political log-rolling. (The child was mentioned in section 2.6.1.)

In this case, programing involves reversal of parental selection procedures. They are to set up conditions likely to occasion nondisturbing behavior and reinforce when it occurs, and periodically do so when it is maintained.

3.3.2.6 *Blackmail contingencies*

In blackmail, the victim pays the blackmailer. The victim positively reinforces extortion. The blackmailer negatively reinforces payment: exposure is averted. In interpersonal relations, one member increases the heat until the other yields, as was noted in the earlier discussion of the escalated breeding of increasingly skillful disturbing patterns (section 3.2.1). Nondisturbing behavior was primitive.

Programing in that case involved a *schedule* reversal. Parents were to set up conditions likely to occasion nondisturbing behavior and then gradually increase the behavior requirement for reinforcement. Disturbing behavior was to be reinforced immediately, before it could escalate. Such programing *seems* counter to common sense: disturbing behavior is to be reinforced immediately, and nondisturbing is to wait? However, (a) it was the "sensible" reverse that produced the skillful disturbing repertoires and primitive nondisturbing repertoire, and (b) the trick often is in setting the occasions and handling the consequences. The following example is illustrative:

> The parents of a [woman of 22 with schizophrenia] reported that she was hallucinating a husband and children at the dinner table and engaging them in extended conversation. If they ignored her (extinction), they knew she would escalate (e.g., hallucinate pregnancy, etc.) until they were forced to reply. If they were punitive, she might start screaming or might stay away from the table and undo their intense efforts to get her there. If they agreed or inquired after the "family" (reinforcement) this, too, might escalate the pattern. ... [The question to be asked was:] what is there about [the hallucinatory patterns] that can be reinforced: most 22 year old women are married, and neighboring daughters were no exception. Her mother said, next time: "Sally, you don't know how delighted I am to hear you considering marriage just like ____ and ____. Believe me, nothing would make father and me happier than ... , etc. ... and that's why we're doing ____ and ____ to make that day come sooner." The parents had to be as ingenious as their daughter in changing the words as they retained the theme to keep up with her changing presentations of the same theme (she had had considerably more experience). By the third week,

hallucinations were replaced by conversations with the existent family. What the parents said was true, and she was treated with honest responses that respected her dignity and also moved the program along.

(Goldiamond, 1974, pp. 51–52)

3.3.2.7 Garbage patterns

Where schedules require high rates of pecking or bar-pressing, the force of each behavior decreases. High rates can be obtained in a variety of other ways, including stimulants, schedule-induction, and presentation of occasions with such history. If muscular effort is then minimized, other efforts may also be. One may recite words with common sounds or sentences with common themes. Efforts to "make sense" of these, if at high rates, may make equal sense. Their sense derives from requirements to behave that exceed the available contingencies.

Negative talk admirably meets these requirements. The set of exclusive statements typically contains many more elements than the set of inclusive statements (a journal is not the *Archives of this*, or *Bulletin of that*, etc.). Rapid or continual verbal behavior can then readily be obtained. It quickly ties into available contingencies when it is turned on listeners in the form of descriptions of their deficiencies; by careful observation, the speaker can zero in on those that score and hone this skill. In interpersonal communication, such behavior is designated as pathological and results in contingency relations of the types discussed, among others. In academic communications, it is often designated as criticism and is reinforced.

Since the types and sources are varied, no general programing procedures hold. The high rate may be attenuated in a variety of ways, including pharmaceutical procedures, contingency elements that attenuate behavior, and contingencies that harness the behavior, that is, that make work for the idling hands, thereby relieving the devil of this task.

3.3.2.8 Outbreak matrices

Psychotic outbreaks have often been assumed to be irrational and nonconsequential outbursts. However, the breaks, like other patterns under discussion, may have been meticulously programed by the environment. At times, it is the culmination of a series of escalating steps and serves to move the person into arrangements preferable to the present ones.[5] One patient took a lethal overdose of drugs and was immediately rushed to the hospital by her succubus husband. Thereafter, he continually held vigil over the ward exit. During a lunch break, and with the aid of her parents, she made her escape to their home.

An even more dramatic case was that of a female paraplegic who had married a man so objectionable to her parents that they had disowned her. The previous year she had pointed a pistol to her chest, and the bullet had entered her spine rather than her heart. She was determined to return to her parents and not to her husband and was making little progress because she had little to do with the therapies available. The staff was wondering into whose hands she could be discharged. The patient took matters into her own hands. She denounced the hairdressers who came in once a week as part of a Mafia conspiracy and spread this information. No one acted on this. The following week she attached a sign to the back of her wheelchair. It read: "Don't blow for the commies. Hitler and Eichmann were right but didn't finish the job." This was written notification; it was written into the nursing chart. Some of the psychologists said all this was just talk and she could be given scissors for the grooming she liked.

The institution not having "listened" early in the escalation process, the patient now forced its hand. That Thursday, when the ward door was wide open and "luckily" when three male attendants were passing by, she was observed bending over the bed of an aphasic patient, a pair of sharp scissors in her upraised hand, stabbing at the patient. She was, of course, instantly seized and transferred to the nearest mental hospital. This is not the end of the story. Her parents took her back (Goldiamond, 1976c, pp. 105–106).

In other cases, the spouse or other members of the family are alerted to what can happen again if they persist in their misbehavior toward that family member. The out*burst* or out*break* (interesting words) may come under other contingency control, as well. I recall one patient who was violent throughout the hour (her alimony payments had not been made), throwing books to the floor, knocking off the papers on my desk, and speaking abusively. However, a relay rack near my desk, with expensive electronic gadgetry, was untouched. Apparently, there was some environmental selection of the targets of the "uncontrolled" rage. Yet another patient, whose constant demands for attention (the call light outside her door was on 20 times a day) the staff suddenly decided to ignore, *did* knock down the color-television set and thereby reinstated the program the staff had dropped.

Outbreaks often involve metaphorical components (matrix c). If the patient talks lucidly during the outbreak or otherwise behaves in a manner interpreted as "normal control," the patient would not obtain the ensuing benefits. Indeed, the costs might be high. Behaving in a manner so that the outburst is labeled as a "psychotic break" may attenuate the costs and provide the benefits (cf. psychotic murder), and such labeling becomes essential to the matrix.

3.3.2.9 Choice of symptoms

The same class of disturbing behaviors can meet the descriptive criteria of different elements of the typology sketched, and different classes of disturbing behaviors can meet the descriptive criteria of any single element in the topology sketched. For example, stuttering can preempt the learning of alternative patterns of social interaction, can fill the speaking space and buy time for formulation of an answer, or can be used in a blackmail contingency, among others. Similarly, a blackmail contingency can be implemented by depressed withdrawal, by aggression, by hallucinating, by the stuttering noted. Such observations (of "secondary gain" to the psychoanalyst) have led to formulation of the following question: what governs symptom choice by a patient? The complex answers given are cut through by the evolutionary restatement: what governs symptom selection by the environment? As it does in other cases, the environment will reinforce a variety of *available* patterns, and the next environment will tend to select a variety from among the then-more probable, and so on, to shape a disturbing behavior directionally. Thus, the parents of one child whose speech is affected by organic trauma may act concerned and sympathetic when this occurs, and the parents of a child in a similar situation are sympathetic when this occurs but speak encouragingly when speech is normal. One environment selects for disturbing behavior and the other selects for an alternative.

Organic patterns may be selected and programed as symptoms. Thus, one patient complained that she blushed constantly and to such an extent that people noticed that she was embarrassed and changed their conversations. This means of control was selected by the environment: the speakers changed their conversations when she blushed and not when other patterns occurred. Vascular changes had always been evident in her skin: it was the "thin" skin often accompanying red hair, and the availability of such changes made them ideal targets for environmental breeding. (Programing involved sensitizing her to such change immediately: "Your skin is more sensitive to the embarrassing trend of a conversation than your ears are. *Listen to your skin.* The instant it starts to warm up, listen to the conversation carefully and start to change it then.") A child who had been sluggish all his life was given Ritalin to activate him. He had no close friends, and other repertoires were limited.

Garbage behavior was produced, and he was hospitalized for a "psychotic outbreak." The ward attendants exhibited concern when he behaved like other patients there, and schizophrenic patterns were rapidly imitated and established.

A symptom that is selected and shaped by the environment into a sophisticated pattern may thus be organic, as well as behavioral. The burgeoning of a biofeedback technology makes it unnecessary to elaborate programing of organicity (cf. Brady and Harris, 1977). Such symptoms may function as operants in the same manner that the more readily observable behavior operants do. The fact that environmental control over organicity can be instated through contingencies into which biofeedback enters should not lead us to the assumption that biofeedback is essential to environmental contingency control over organicity. Programed biofeedback merely systematizes what has been going on for a long time, just as *p.i.* systematizes book instruction and *p.s.i.* classroom instruction. And, these technologies being new, they have been applied only to a small fraction of the vast areas they systematize. Just as one can teach classes effectively without this technology, one can alter patient organicity similarly. Indeed, other environments have been programing patient organicity for some time, and patients may have been selecting the conditions that do so over others that do not in accord with a contingency matrix. If a headache will serve as a convenient social operant, a practiced person can nurse it along from origins that could have been programed into other directions, as well.

It can be argued that biological evolution selects for behavior and thereby for the organs involved, as readily as stating that evolution selects for organs that thereby permit behavior.[6] And this may hold as well for environmental resolution of a contingency matrix into which organicity enters and the consequent programing of organicity. Certainly, in general medicine, major organic problems are attributed to persistent behavior patterns and are therefore governed by the social environment. One example is the behavior of smoking, with its attendant effects on cancer and cardiac arrest. Smoking has been considered an addiction and therefore under organic control, Drive→B. However, anyone who has smoked heavily knows that very few of the cigarettes smoked belong in the relief-from-craving category. Heavy smokers know they smoke but don't know why. And compulsive eaters are not continually hungry. These behaviors of medical significance require fine-grain contingency analysis. Such patterns of behavior, among others, can produce organic change that, given our present knowledge, is irreversible. Ensuing environmental selection of behavior may then program from a different base.

3.4 Programs for mental health/illness

That the contingencies that govern the disturbing behaviors of the mentally ill are to be found governing the behaviors of anyone else should be evident upon rereading the incomplete typology presented. Nor would a more complete typology alter this. To cite but a few examples from the contingencies of everyday academic life:

1. *Social matrices.* College enrollment may increase during depression for those who can afford it, and who have academic skills, for reasons similar to increase in mental hospital enrollment for those who cannot afford college enrollment, and who have skills in using the public system.
2. *Individual matrices.* Some academics publish profusely and find little good to write about their colleagues; they are promoted (for critical acumen) and thereby enhance and maintain their community standing, in contingencies similar to those governing the destructive verbal behavior of the obsessional patient who maintained her community standing thereby.

3. *Matrices involving metaphors.* Reading abstruse material and getting paid for thinking about it is sanctioned by attaching an academic label and, in a similar contingency, being fearful of cockroaches and getting concerned attention for being immobilized by it is sanctioned by attaching a psychiatric label. The reader may complete the remaining contingencies, using observations in academia or elsewhere. Such scenarios, of course, are not devoid of emotion.

By centering my discussion on rationalization of contingencies, I have paid very little attention to the affect accompanying the contingencies. However, as was noted earlier (Chapter 2, section 2.4.1, "Emotions, behaviors, and contingencies"), affect or emotions are not excluded from the system. Indeed, since affect can often suggest the presence of a contingency that is not apparent from content, its expression is explicitly solicited in at least one type of programing ("treatment") derived from the radical behaviorist model (Goldiamond, 1974, pp. 37, 74, 81, 82). The effort here is often to *sensitize* patients to their own private affect as a guide to the burgeoning public contingencies they might then try to forestall or strengthen while the contingencies may be malleable.

Because the behavior of patients is considered to be rational does not imply that the patients are happy or are not miserable. The ascription of rationality simply states that a model that rationalizes the matrix contingencies adequately describes the data. The child whose disturbing behavior produces parental concern (which would not occur otherwise) in the form of nagging and punishment (section 3.3.2.5, "Mutual disturbance") is *resentful* when he is stopped, and the parent whose nagging and punishment are negatively reinforced by his stopping are *upset* at the time and for some time thereafter. It is their unhappiness with this state of affairs, they report, that occasions their application for help (patients come for treatment "when they're hurting").[7] Stated otherwise, patients *deserve consideration as rational sufferers*, and the suffering may be intense. Labeling them as mentally ill may increase the suffering, but it may provide them access for care and help that our social system would not provide *if they were labeled in any other manner*. As will be noted shortly, this holds for branches of medicine other than psychiatry.

Aid to the suffering and relief of their distress has long been considered a humane and noble undertaking, and much of the reverence for medicine as a calling derives from its association with this undertaking of help. In this task, diagnosis of a particular pathology (*paqos*, Gr., suffering, disease; *logos*, Gr., word, discourse) plays a critical role. It implies a particular course that the disease will follow and a particular therapy (*qerapein*, Gr., healing). The field of mental illness continues with the humane undertaking. Here, too, there is diagnosis of *psycho*pathologies, on the basis of what is wrong or deranged. Among the treatments is psychotherapy. When clinical psychologists, social workers, and others enter the field on the grounds that they are equally capable of diagnosis and psychotherapy, they do so as helping professionals, in the same tradition of humane aid. And when a different approach derived from learning laboratories of experimental psychology enters, it, too, is a helping profession that provides aid for those with behavior disorders, through behavior therapy; the newer clinical psychologists claim similar origins but speak of cognitive disorders and cognitive therapy. The continuity possibly reflects a philosophic continuity that, so to speak, is spoken in the different tongues and manipulations of different disciplines. On the other hand, they may reflect common and pervasive contingencies of our social system.

Before considering what social contingencies may be involved, the existence of a divergent approach should be noted. This approach, too, is concerned with aid to the suffering and relief of their distress and, accordingly, pursues the traditional aims discussed. However, rather than diagnosing for specified pathology, whose elimination (or relief from which) is the outcome, it diagnoses for specified outcome, whose construction (or attainment) is the outcome. A key difference between the two approaches, the pathological and the constructional (Goldiamond, 1974), is the area to which *specificity* is assigned. There is a considerable difference between specifying an obsession or compulsion and specifying particular interpersonal or marital skills. Suffering or distress is eliminated or alleviated in the one by eliminating a pathology and in the other by establishing an outcome. If there is a difference in which area is sharply bounded, there is a corollary difference in the *unbounded area* outside. In the pathological case, health is simply defined as the unbounded area outside of pathology. Substitution of terms such as *health* attainment for *disease* elimination supplies no information not contained in the latter, since it is defined by it. Accordingly, initial assessment must be of the well-bounded set, pathology, rather than of the otherwise undetermined outcome area around it. In the constructional case, the unbounded area is all of the multiple ways in which matrix resolutions can be distressful. Accordingly, initial assessment is not of those multiple ways but rather of what well-bounded outcomes to construct, what current strengths can serve as starting points, what transitional procedures make sense, and what reinforcers to apply. Specificity of constructional outcomes makes possible the formulation of a contract with programing limited to those aims and those aims only. These limitations parallel those found in other contracts, commercial and legal, and in the constitutional contract between the people and their representatives. It is the vagueness of pathologically derived outcomes ("eliminating destructive tendencies") in the mental hospital that rationalizes the substitution of a fiduciary relation for a contractual one and produces tension between constitutionally guaranteed rights of patients and protection of others by incarceration of patients (for a more extended discussion, see Goldiamond, 1974).

An example of a social institution that is mainly constructional is found in the educational system. College students are classified by their "majors" (or "concentrations"), and graduate and professional students by their degree programs or professions. Students whose deficits differ sit in classes whose communality is governed by the specific outcome stated in the catalog. Unfortunately, the effort to attain this is too often equated with the preparation of an outline assumed to produce it, and students are expected to fail. In *p.i.*, and *p.s.i.*, the program has been tested through meticulously kept records that have helped assess functional relations between program interventions and specified student behavior outcomes. Such assessment continues. Students are not failed. What is recorded is the point at which they stop. They may resume at that point at some later time. The educational system, for all its pathologies, has been able to reconcile mass institutions and individualized outcomes. This it does by having a variety of outcome "packets," each listed in the college catalog (and each of which is broken up into smaller packets). The packets can be lectures, demonstrations, group sessions, etc. The student's individual curriculum is specified by which combinations of packets are selected. Although the offering may be standard (in *p.i.* they are also tailored), theoretically, decades may pass before one student repeats the curriculum of another. In the field of mental health, such usable packets are being developed for the establishment of differentiating skills, but, at present, these are dictated by the needs or populations of a particular investigator. No statement is made that systematized development of *p.c.i.* (programed clinical intervention) will solve all problems; the educational system certainly allows for considerable individual professor–student interaction and ravel programs. Certainly there are a variety of basic living skills that should not have to be retaught for almost every patient, as most psychotherapists will admit. The development of such packets could flow from present practice – if practitioners kept records of operant precision, relating the fine grain of their interventions to the fine-grain of the referent patient behavior and the fine grain of other controlling environments. The *practice* of medicine (as distinguished from its best-articulated ideology; see below) supplies one example. Meticulous records close to the type discussed are kept. And the attending physicians do not mix every medicine themselves: they prescribe medicines and treatment from available stocks and other personnel. Occasionally, there is a laying-on of hands. The practice of *p.i.–p.s.i.–p.c.i.* and its radical behaviorist rationale (which specifies the fine grains of the governing contingencies) is probably the closest working example.

It should not be assumed that medical (including psychiatric) *practice* is governed in its entirety by the pathological orientation. For some time, and increasingly, the profession has been applying constructional outcomes (to produce functioning of a specified type), assessing current strengths, and so on, in meticulously well-formulated programs. These include detailed records to help assess functional relations between medical interventions and the specified patient outcomes toward which the interventions were directed. What is involved, then, is the existence of a variety of medical models. However, the pathological model is, at present, the most precisely articulated one. Rhetoric directed against *the* medical model logically rests on misassumed congruence between medicine and this model. And this model has had so extraordinary a staying power that it has been extended to other areas, e.g., social pathology, with all its symptoms.

NOTES

1   "Wa" at one age will be reinforced socially and by water. At a later age, "wa-wa" may so be required. And at yet a later date, "water" and "want water," etc.

2   A graduate student, who was driving a university station wagon on which "Committee on Evolutionary Biology" plainly appeared, stopped for gasoline at a station in Kansas. The owner's wife then asked: "Tell me son, have you seen any evolution going on?"

3   The behaviors need not be shaped. They may exist in the repertoire in different contingencies, and the task becomes to transfer such control. A patient had never invited guests to dinner because she didn't know how – her mother had been a recluse and had never had guests. The patient had, however, successfully directed television shows in which guests on opposing sides of controversial issues talked. She was told to treat her dinner guests like talk-show guests – seat neutrals between them at the table, etc.

4   A moral outcry may then be heard: "You shouldn't pay people to get well!" This misses the economic point that such payment may be less than the costs attached to disturbing behavior.

5   The statement can also be <u>out</u> of the present arrangements. However, research on children who run <u>away</u> from home has found that they generally run <u>to</u> specific places, and apprehension of AWOLs in the Army has generally been aided by assigning agents to the places they are likely to run <u>to</u>.

6   When, for example, reflected light is a condition under which one pattern of behavior produces consequences that another pattern does not, the environment may thereby select organisms with a cluster of photosensitive cells. There will be behavioral differences among such offspring, and the environment may then select the more complex over less complex cluster, and so on, over thousands of generations. It is not that the mammalian eye permits skilled behavior, but possibly that skilled behavior requires a mammalian eye.

7   Applying <u>for</u> treatment is operant behavior. However, the contingency specified (Ap→Tr) may be part of a metaphorical matrix. It may rationalize disturbing behavior ("I don't know what gets into me when I act this way, I must be sick"). It may also sanction disturbing behavior ("I don't know (etc.) … , but you get worse before you get better"), get the person out of difficulties ("I promised the judge I'd seek treatment"), be used punitively ("You've made me so upset that I'm seeing a shrink"), produce control ("I'm not going to tell you what we talked about"), be used to gain an ally ("And not only did they yell at me, but …"), and to provide other consequences, among which, of course, is the help requested.

4

Societal contingencies
of the pathology model

4.1 THE INDIVIDUAL SOCIAL SELECTION PARALLEL

The relation between social ideology and social movements has been debated for some time. Do ideologies produce movements; movements, ideologies; or do both go together? In parallel with earlier discussions on the relation of behavior to emotions, awareness, conceptualization, purpose, and decisions, I shall advance the argument that social ideology and social movements are both governed by social contingencies in different functional relations, that one can occur without the other or precede it, and that over the long run, changes in both will reflect changes in contingencies.[1] Accordingly, I shall present some evidence that bears on this argument and then consider the contingencies governing a few ideologies in mental health/illness.

The case study will be that of *p.i.*: Skinner's *Science* (1958) article brought teaching machines and their rationale to the attention of an important audience. The article was one of several on teaching, and especially teaching of science. The National Defense Education Act was enacted that year. Educational theories and systems were being discussed, and legislative action was taken. Their governing relation may have not been to each other but rather to the fact that the Russians had penetrated space the previous year, with Sputnik I followed by Sputnik II. The consequence toward which American policy was shifted was American superiority. This was contingent on the production of scientific manpower and support of training and education. NASA was founded. The social contingencies seem clear.

These particular contingencies were not responsible for *p.i.*, which was an educational extension of a radical behaviorism ("system of thought, ideology") hitherto related to laboratory animal research. What the social system did in 1958 and thereafter was to make available increased financial support for such research; further funding was made contingent on progress reports. The social system increased the probability of hitherto low probability educational behavior – it reinforced, selected, or bred in that direction.[2]

Since that time, such selection has shaped *p.i.* into a variety of novel forms. A recognizable mutation in the form of *p.s.i.* has been reinforced to the point that "about 2,000 [*p.s.i.*] courses are being given each semester" at more than one hundred colleges and universities, according to a *Sunday Times* article headlined by: "Self-Paced Instruction. An Innovation That Stuck" (Miller, 1977, p. 9).

The parallel of selection by the social system to evolutionary selection and individual contingency programing is evident: "The statement, 'There is nothing as powerful as an

DOI: 10.4324/9781003260103-4

idea whose time has come' translates into the power of an 'idea which rationalizes contingencies whose time has come'" (Goldiamond, 1974, p. 116).

4.2 CONTINGENCIES OF PATHOLOGICAL IDEOLOGY AND ALTERNATIVES

A system of thought and behavior as powerful as the pathological model obviously is governed by widespread and recurrent social contingencies. Accordingly, my discussion will be limited to a small segment of these.

4.2.1 Consulting room contingencies

Until recently, the major setting for modern Western medicine was the consulting room or home; hospitals were extensions of these. Individual patients paid individual physicians for services. Third-party payment merely substitutes for the individual, and to the extent that the federal government enters, short of socialized medicine, the tradition will continue. Psychologists and other nonmedical mental health professionals are now actively campaigning for "Freedom of Choice" legislation to extend impending federal payment to their private treatment, and among such professionals are those with a behavioral orientation.

Where the patient (or patient-surrogates) pays the practitioner for services, the services must be for the patient (or designee). The problem to be solved, then, is most likely to be an individual *problem*, that is, one centered in the patient. The patient is mentally ill, or exhibits psychopathology, or exhibits disturbed or disordered behavior. And the problem is then the patient's mind, psyche, or conditioning history. Such analysis is easy to adapt to a pathological model with prestige and standing and presumably then taps the same supporting social contingencies.

Those who have followed the history of behavior modification will observe one major deviation from the consulting room and from the pathological model. It was in various state institutions for children with cognitive disabilities, and in state mental hospitals for adults, that the constructional model derived from radical behaviorist work first received application to clinical problems. The aim was to construct new repertoires for the cognitively disabled, teach language to the mute, etc., and, similarly, to construct or reinstate repertoires for living outside for the mentally ill. *The professionals involved were on the state payroll.* They were not being paid by the patients for services to them. (This is a later development.) And it is of interest that in the state institutions for the cognitively disabled, at least where they were given free access (this was typically not the case in mental hospitals) and developed constructional delivery systems, they were able to succeed where the pathological systems had failed.

The relation of socioeconomic contingencies to treatment ideologies seems clear, in these two cases.

4.2.2 Patient support contingencies

Yet another mainstay of the pathological model has been the withdrawal of social support for the patient if the problem is not stated in terms of pathological treatment. For example, one rehabilitation hospital set up third-way (as opposed to halfway) houses for patients: they could progressively move through them and toward home as their rehabilitation progressed. The costs would become progressively cheaper as medical–hospital involvement diminished. Third-party payment was withdrawn for stages outside the regular hospital. The physiatrists (physical medicine physicians), faced with no financial support of patients for improvement through the third-way system, kept patients hospitalized.

A newspaper article that would be whimsical, did it not have overtones of the type described, refers to the establishment of the second American hospital center for *gambling*. Indeed, the legalization of gambling is compared to spread of pneumonia. "Everyone in this room could contract pneumonia, so you wouldn't bring someone with pneumonia into the room and sneeze," a psychologist is quoted as saying. The gambler, like the alcoholic (but see Keehn reference earlier), requires admission to a "hospital to detoxify, where he could become seriously ill or die if he doesn't receive attention"; the hospital is necessary to "cope with the more profound emotional problems that compulsive gambling usually masks" (the quotations are from psychologists). Gamblers get very little sustained professional concern. A psychiatrist notes that "psychiatrists don't like these people. They lie, they require endless buttering up. ... And besides, they don't pay their bills" (Slavin, 1977, p. 35).

The contingency issue raised by the article is that social support is provided only if the behavior patterns involved are assigned a pathological label. Hence, the possibly forthcoming designation of "pathological gambling" as a psychiatric problem in the forthcoming Diagnostic and Statistical Manual of the American Psychiatric Association would be "[a] significant step forward" (Slavin, 1977, p. 35). While such pathology-contingent support may maintain socially undesirable professional patterns and undesirable patient patterns, it may also maintain some desirable support for the sufferer and, therefore, for professionals. The labeling issue is by no means one-sided. An alternative strategy might be to attempt to provide *social support for constructional programs*, that is, those that do not label the person as mentally ill, or behaviorally disordered, but consider patients to be rational sufferers who require constructional outcomes. Such a social turnabout would also serve to orient professional behavior into constructional research and programing.

4.2.3 Labeling contingencies

There are other issues involved in labeling. As was noted earlier, the campuses of mental hospitals could be used to train and establish living skills through constructionally oriented programs. Instead, hospitals are being dismantled. Similarly, rehabilitation hospitals are denounced as producing isolation from society, instead of returning patients to the mainstream. However, such stay as noted earlier may be governed by the social system rather than the professionals involved. Further, these institutions, like mental hospitals, can serve to protect families that might otherwise be shattered by the requirements of a mental patient or a severely handicapped person. A question that might be asked is "how might the institutions be better used?" Slogans directed against institutionalization and "warehousing of the mentally ill" simply serve to justify the dismemberment, as do catchwords like "mainstreaming."

What is involved, of course, is the matrix resolution of various societal alternatives, and competing and intersecting requirements of different social subsystems. Care is still needed for the handicapped, and someone must bear the costs, but in "mainstreaming," the costs may be simply transferred from the public to the private sector, possibly the family. And custodial care for the mentally ill in some "convalescent-centers" *seems* to be less costly than institutions engaged in programing living skills. However, the benefits of the latter would appear to be greater. To assume that a decision matrix is being ignored is to ignore the fact that agencies providing the funds for custody or programing are usually not the ones getting the financial benefits. Agency behavior is then not irrational. Nor should it be assumed that the social system is inept. The task is to make explicit the contingency matrices operating, for the competing social systems as it is for the individual. And social analysts often simply supply rhetoric that diverts attention from the contingencies operating and from cost transfers between federal, state, local, and various private sectors (cf. Miller, 1977).

4.2.4 Contingencies supporting cross-directional movement

Where consulting-room practice has been successful, this has by and large been with individual problems. Successful treatment is possible here in two cases: (a) where the problem is individual, as in the individual matrices discussed previously (Chapter 3, section 3.3.2.4, "The preempted deficit"), or (b) where the problem is individual, but its origin resides in widespread environmental conditions, social or otherwise. An individual addict may be taught other ways, and a cancer patient might be helped, but it is more economical to treat the environmental condition, as public health has done. Nevertheless, the suffering patient can be helped – but more will keep coming. However, individual treatment will be ineffective under those conditions (c) where the individual problem is a function of social variables. The patient whose impending disability settlement was contingent on magnitude of disability was an example. In other cases, payments for living at home (and following a health maintenance regimen) are often minimal when compared to payments and support when the person is ill (has not followed the regimen). In such cases, "deterioration is being programmed" (Goldiamond, 1976b, p. 130). Such patients, regardless of "attitude," present the professional with an almost unmanageable problem. Here, it is the widespread contingencies that first require change.

Increasing concern is being expressed over the limitations of individually based elimination of pathology, the category (a) above, which has been a mainstay of this model. At present, the concern is mainly heard in general medicine, about which such questions are asked as: has biological treatment reached its limits, and is the increasing cost of such treatment at all matched by a similar increase in cure rate? Or, should medicine move away from the biological model and become a social science? In cardiac arrest, the suspect variables are smoking, cholesterol, and hypertension. All of these involve patterns of behavior outside, with extensive support from the social system. And yet, another case seems presented by diseases such as diabetes. If patients could monitor signs outside and engage in appropriate living habits, they might stay out of the hospital for longer periods of time, and when they report, report *on time*, when the problem is more amenable to change.

The chronic handling of such patients poses problems for general medicine. First, its practitioners are not trained in the behavior-contingency analysis treatment required. Second, their orientation is toward medical delivery in hospitals, rather than programing delivery outside. Third, the reward system in which they have practiced is of immediate reinforcement of professional intervention. Long-term effects and chronic care are mainly reserved for psychiatry and the very few who go into physiatry. However, the meticulous programing procedures of radical behaviorists do provide reinforcement at each step for the programer, just as they do for the learner, and their meticulousness parallels recorded intervention in medicine. (See Goldiamond, 1975a, pp. 29–32 for further discussion of this point.) In all events, general medicine is becoming increasingly attentive to interventions hitherto not associated with medicine. Its theorists are becoming similarly attentive to nonbiological variables (Engel, 1977).

Simultaneously, much of psychiatry is moving in the opposite direction, with increasing emphasis on biological intervention and biological theory. As I have noted elsewhere:

> Given the competition for the tax dollar, federal and state agencies are increasingly becoming concerned about what they are getting for their money. This issue is also being raised by

consumer groups. … Psychiatrists, of course, in common with other medical colleagues, can offer chemotherapies and other intrusive organic interventions. And these yield to cost–benefit analyses more readily than psychotherapy. Psychiatrists, accordingly, are increasingly stressing the drug-prescription approach they share with the rest of medical practice. They thereby assert their rights to inclusion in what are, after all, health programs, as defined in the context of medical insurance.

(Goldiamond, 1976d, p. 146)

And, we should expect growing emphasis and support of theory (ideology) that assigns mental illness to biological or genetic variables. Nothing in the foregoing should be interpreted as opposition to the acquisition of such knowledge, or to appropriate pharmacologic intervention, since it can serve expeditiously as part of a treatment program, pathological or constructional (e.g., Goldiamond and Dyrud, 1968). I am merely reiterating the relation of societal contingencies to professional behavior *and* ideology (theory). It should be noted that this psychiatric trend toward organic interpretation may relate to a socially required closer identification with the intervention procedures of general medicine, *as medicine is presently defined.* Such definition is within a biomedical context, which can accept mental illness most readily when the *illness* is interpreted literally. However, the same economic considerations that govern increasing study of cost-effectiveness and thereby the accompanying movement to psychiatric interventions of a biomedical type also govern *increased attentiveness to societal interventions.* And these economic contingencies may also govern *movement toward more socially oriented theories* (ideologies) and away from the present definitions of medicine, pathology, and illness, with their biomedical referents.

4.2.5 L'envoi

Some societal contingencies may already be available to mesh with constructional approaches. Professionals can be considered double agents, serving both their clients and the societal system that licenses or certifies them and supports them in other ways. Where the outcomes of the individual are consonant with those of the social system (the patient "desires" to get back to work, and the social system also "desires" this), and the professionals hired by both as the change agent do not produce the necessary change, then, perhaps, professionals may turn to alternative models of intervention and the related alternative ideologies. Perhaps such gradual change will bring about the shift – if the systems are responsive, and if the constructional approach has something to contribute, and if its practitioners are engaged in contribution.

An alternative or supplementary task is possible. At present, economic and other contingencies are geared to support pathological orientations and labeling. Indeed, economic support of change is withdrawn when intervention is nonmedical, as biologically defined. The supplementary task, then, is to redefine the science and discipline of medicine to *include* variables and approaches other than the individual-organic. The inclusion of such variables makes it possible, at the very least, to have alternatives whose various outcomes we can compare with those produced by the pathological model. Rather than rhetoric in this area, and rather than arguments in support of one approach over another, it would seem that data are needed on the costs, benefits, and efforts for the various alternative societal policies available. Among the social models that lend themselves to explicit analysis is the constructional programing model that has been the subject of this discussion.

Setting up a decision matrix for our various options does not guarantee, of course, that the decision rules that rationalize the matrix are to our liking. However, it might make evident what rules are being applied, and this is a first step.

I address myself to medicine because impending federal entry into the societal contingency matrix is being rationalized in terms of health. Much of medicine is already constructional. And much of psychiatry and physiatry, among other specialties, is concerned with contingency-change, implicitly if not explicitly. Public health is concerned with environmental intervention and is considering such life-style behaviors as smoking and inappropriate food ingestion to be public health problems; focus is on establishment of alternative behavioral styles in these areas. And nonmedical professions and consumers' groups are making known their demands. These portents may be coincidental. However, they may suggest changing societal contingencies in search of a rationalizing ideology to replace or supplement the pathological one. I herewith nominate a constructional programing approach.

NOTES

1   This discussion is condensed from "The professional as a double-agent" (Goldiamond, 1978).

2   One difference should be made between ideology-movement and awareness-behavior. Ideologies are observable patterns: their points are printed, circulated, and argued. Emotions, etc., are private events. What may be at issue in an ideology-movement discussion is two different patterns of observable behaviors of individuals, with each individual exhibiting ideological and political behaviors that seem similar to those of other individuals (although on close observation of tribal ceremonies, J. A. Jones [1977] reports, the contingencies of each participant's behavior are often different). Nevertheless, ideology is reflected by individual "consciousness raising," to use the current idiom, and the analogy to awareness becomes apt.

References

Azrin, N. H. (1958). Some effects of noise on human behavior. *Journal of the Experimental Analysis of Behavior, 1*, 183–200.

Azrin, N. H., Hake, D. F., & Hutchinson, R. R. (1965). Elicitation of aggression by a physical blow. *Journal of the Experimental Analysis of Behavior, 8*, 55–57.

Azrin, N. H., Hutchinson, R. R., & Hake, D. F. (1966). Extinction-induced aggression. *Journal of the Experimental Analysis of Behavior, 9*, 191–201.

Azrin, N. H., Hutchinson, R. R., & McLaughlin, R. (1965). The opportunity for aggression as an operant reinforcer during aversive stimulation. *Journal of the Experimental Analysis of Behavior, 8*, 171–180.

Azrin, N. H., Hutchinson, R. R., & Sallery, R. D. (1964). Pain-aggression toward inanimate objects. *Journal of the Experimental Analysis of Behavior, 7*, 223–228.

Becker, G. S., & Landes, W. H. (Eds.) (1974). *Essays in the economics of crime and punishment*. New York: National Bureau of Economic Research.

Becker, H. S. (1963). *Outsiders: studies in the sociology of deviance*. New York: Free Press.

Bell, R. Q. (1974). Contributions of human infants to caregiving and social interaction. In M. Lewis & L. A. Rosenblum (Eds.), *The effect of the infant on its caregiver*. New York: John Wiley & Sons.

Brady, J. V., & Harris, A. (1977). The experimental production of altered physiological states. In W. K. Honig & J. E. R. Staddon (Eds.), *Handbook of operant behavior*. Englewood Cliffs, NJ: Prentice-Hall.

Braginsky, B. M., Braginsky, D. D., & Ring, K. (1969). *Methods of madness: the mental hospital as a last resort*. New York: Holt, Rinehart & Winston.

Caggiula, A. R. (1972). Shock-elicited copulation and aggression in male rats. *Journal of Comparative & Physiological Psychology, 80*, 393–397.

Caggiula. A. R., & Eibergen, R. (1969). Copulation of virgin male rats evoked by painful peripheral stimulation. *Journal of Comparative Physiological Psychology, 69*, 414–419.

Collier, G. F., & Somfay, S. A. (1974). *Ascent from Skid Row: the Bon Accord community – 1961–1973*. Toronto: Addiction Research Foundation of Ontario.

Day, W. (1969). Radical behaviorism in reconciliation with phenomenology. *Journal of the Experimental Analysis of Behavior, 12*, 315–328.

Delgado, J. M. R. (1969). *Physical control of the mind: toward a psychocivilized society*. New York: Harper E. Row.

Egan, J. P. (1975). *Signal detection theory and ROC analysis*. New York: Academic Press.

Engel, G. L. (1977). The need for a new medical model: a challenge for biomedicine. *Science, 196*, 129–136.

Fairweather, G. W., Sanders, D. H., Maynard, H., & Cressler, D. L. (1969). *Community life for the mentally ill: an alternative to institutional care*. Chicago: Aldine.

Falk, J. L. (1961). Production of polydipsia in normal rats by an intermittent food schedule. *Science, 133*, 195–196.

Garner, W. R., Hake, H. W., & Eriksen, C. W. (1956). Operationism and the concept of perception. *Psychological Review, 63*(3), 149–159.

Gilbert, R. M. (1970). Psychology and biology. *Canadian Psychologist, 11*, 221–238.

Gilbert, R. M., & Keehn, J. O. (Eds.) (1972). *Schedule effects: drugs, drinking, and aggression*. Toronto: University of Toronto.

Goldiamond, I. (1959). The hysteria over subliminal advertising as a misunderstanding of science. *American Psychologist, 14*, 398–599.

Goldiamond, I. (1962). Perception. In A. J. Bachrach (Ed.), *Experimental foundations of clinical psychology*. New York: Basic Books.

Goldiamond, I. (1964). Response bias in perceptual communication. *Disorders of Communication* 42, Chapter 23. Research Publications, Association for Research in Nervous and Mental Diseases.

Goldiamond, I. (1965a). Stuttering and fluency as manipulatable operant response classes. In L. Krasner & P. Ullmann (Eds.), *Research in behavior modification*. New York: Holt, Rinehart & Winston.

Goldiamond, I. (1965b). Self-control procedures in personal behavior problems. *Psychological Reports Monograph*, *17*(3), 851–68.

Goldiamond, I. (1966). Perception, language, and conceptualization rules. In B. Kleinmuntz (Ed.), *Problem solving*. New York: John Wiley & Sons.

Goldiamond. I. (1974). Toward a constructional approach to social problems: ethical and constitutional issues raised by applied behavior analysis. *Behaviorism*, *2*(1), 1–84.

Goldiamond, I. (1975a). Alternative sets as a framework for behavioral formulations and research. *Behaviorism*, *3*(1), 49–86.

Goldiamond, I. (1975b). Singling out behavior modification for legal regulation: some effects on patient care, psychotherapy, and research in general. *Arizona Law Review*, *17*, 105–126.

Goldiamond, I. (1976a). Protection of human subjects and patients: a social contingency analysis of distinctions between research and practice, and its implications. *Behaviorism*, *4*(1), 1–41.

Goldiamond, I. (1976b). Self-reinforcement. *Journal of Applied Behavior Analysis*, *9*, 509–514.

Goldiamond, I. (1976c). Coping and adaptive behaviors of the disabled. In G. L. Albrecht (Ed.), *The sociology of physical illness and rehabilitation*. Pittsburgh: University of Pittsburgh.

Goldiamond, I. (1976d). Singling out self-administered behavior therapies for professional overview: a comment on Rosen. *American Psychologist*, *31*(2), 142–147.

Goldiamond, I. (1977). Insider–outsider problems: a constructional approach. *Rehabilitation Psychology*, *22*, 103–116.

Goldiamond, I. (1978). The professional as a double-agent. *Journal of Applied Behavior Analysis*, *11*(1), 178–184.

Goldiamond, I., & Dyrud, J. E. (1968). Some applications and implications of behavioral analysis for psychotherapy. In J. Schlien (Ed.), *Research in Psychotherapy* 3. Washington, DC: American Psychological Association.

Green, D. M., & Swets, J. A. (1966). *Signal detection theory and psychophysics*. New York: John Wiley & Sons.

Hayes, S. C., & Barlow, D. H. (1977). The scope of behavior modification. Paper delivered at the Annual Convention, Association for the Advancement of Behavior Therapy, Atlanta, GA, Dec. 7–10, 1977.

Hefferline, R. F., Keenan, B., & Harford, R. (1959). Escape and avoidance conditioning in human subjects without their observation of the response. *Science*, *130*, 1338–1339.

Hendershot, C. N. (1967). *Programmed learning: a bibliography of programs and presentation devices*. Bay City, MI: Hendershot (Supplements 1967, 1968, 1969).

Hendershot, C. N. (1973). *Programmed learning and individually paced instruction*. Bay City, MI: Hendershot.

Heston, L. L. (1966). Psychiatric disorders in foster home reared children of schizophrenic mothers. *British Journal of Psychiatry*, *112*, 819–825.

Hilgard, E. R. (1948). *Theories of learning*. New York: Appleton-Century-Crofts.

Hilgard, E. R., & Bower, G. H. (1966). *Theories of learning* (3rd ed.). New York: Appleton-Century-Crofts.

Holland. J. G., & Skinner, B. F. (1961). *The analysis of behavior*. New York: McGraw-Hill.

Holz, C., & Azrin, N. H. (1961). Discriminative properties of punishment. *Journal of the Experimental Analysis of Behavior*, *4*, 225–232.

Hutchinson, R. R. (1977). Byproducts of aversive control. In J. R. Honig & J. E. R. Staddon (Eds.), *Handbook of operant behavior*. Englewood Cliffs, NJ: Prentice-Hall.

Jensen, A. R. (1969). How much can we boost IQ and scholastic achievement? *Harvard Educational Review*, *39*, 1–123.

Jones, J. A. (1977, May). *Social reinforcement and social-change*. Paper delivered at the 3rd Annual Convention, Midwest Association of Behavior Analysis, Chicago.

Karp, H. J. (1975). *The effects of consequences on sensitivity to nonfluency: a signal detection approach*. Unpublished doctoral dissertation, Department of Psychology, University of Chicago.

Keehn, J. D. (1976). Schedule-dependent aggression. In E. Ribes-Inesta and A. Bandura (Eds.), *Analysis of delinquency and aggression*. Hillsdale, NJ: Lawrence Erlbaum Associates.

Keehn, J. D., Kuechier, N. A., Oki, G., Collier, G., & Walsh, R. (1973). Interpersonal behaviorism and community treatment of alcoholics. *Proceedings of the First Annual Alcoholism Conference of the National Institute on Alcohol Abuse and Alcoholism: Research on Alcoholism: Clinical Problems and Special Populations*. Rockville, MD: National Institute of Alcohol Abuse and Alcoholism, NIMH, 153–176.

Keller, F. S., & Schoenfeld, N. N. (1950). *Principles of psychology*. New York: Appleton-Century-Crofts.

Kling, J. N. (1971). Learning: introductory survey. In J. N. Kling & L. A. Riggs (Eds.), *Woodworth and Schlosberg's Experimental Psychology* (3rd ed.). New York: Holt, Rinehart & Winston.

Korner, A. F. (1974). The effects of the infant's state, level of arousal, sex, and ontogenetic stage on the caregiver. In M. Lewis and L. A. Rosenblum (Eds.), *The effect of the infant on its caregiver*. New York: John Wiley & Sons.

Laing, R. D. (1969). *The divided self*. New York: Pantheon (original ed.: 1960).

Lewis, M., & Rosenblum, L. A. (Eds.) (1974). *The effect of the infant on its caregiver.* New York: John Wiley & Sons.

Luce, R. D., & Raiffa. N. (1957). *Games and decisions: introduction and critical survey.* New York: John Wiley & Sons.

Lusted, L. B. (1971). Signal detectability and medical decision-making. *Science, 171,* 1217–1219.

Markle, S. M. (1975). *Good frames and bad* (3rd ed.). Chicago: Tiemann Associates.

Medawar, P. B. (1977, Feb. 3). Unnatural science. *New York Review of Books, 34*(1), 13–18.

Miller, J. (1977, May 1). Self-paced instruction: an innovation that stuck. *New York Times,* sec. 4, p. 9, at 1–4.

Miller, S. M. (1977). Technipol or expert? *Social Policy, 7*(5), 4–6.

Moore, J. (1975). On the principle of operationism in a science of behavior. *Behaviorism, 3*(2), 120–138.

Morse, N. H., & Kelleher, R. T. (1970). Schedules as fundamental determinants of behavior. In N. N. Schoenfeld (Ed.), *The theory of reinforcement schedules.* New York: Appleton-Century-Crofts.

Moss, N. A. (1967). Sex, age, and state as determinants of mother–child interaction. *Merrill-Palmer Quarterly of Behavior and Development, 13*(1), 19–36.

Moss, N. A., & Robson, K. S. (1968). Maternal influences in early social visual behavior. *Child Development, 31,* 401–408.

O'Brien, F., & Azrin, N. H. (1973). Interaction-priming: a method of reinstating patient–family relationships. *Behaviour Research and Therapy, 11,* 133–136.

Paul, J. (1968). The return of punitive sterilization proposals: current attacks on illegitimacy and the AFDC program. *Law and Society Review, 3*(1), 77–106.

Premack, D. (1976). *Intelligence in ape and man.* Hillsdale, NJ: Lawrence Erlbaum Associates.

Rachman, S., & Teasdale, J. (1969). *Aversion therapy and behaviour disorders: an analysis.* Coral Gables, FL: University of Miami.

Rayfield, F., Segal, M., & Goldiamond, I. (1982). Schedule-induced defecation. *Journal of the Experimental Analysis of Behavior, 38,* 19–34.

Rosenthal, D. (1970). *Genetic theory and abnormal behavior.* New York: McGraw-Hill.

Scheff, T. J. (1966). *Being mentally ill: sociological theory.* Chicago: Aldine.

Sidman, M. (1960a). Normal sources of pathological behavior. *Science, 132,* 61.

Sidman, M. (1960b). *Tactics of scientific research: evaluating experimental data in psychology.* New York: Research Press.

Sidman, M., & Stoddard, L. T. (1966). Programming perception and learning for retarded children. *International Review of Research in Mental Retardation, 2,* 151–208.

Sidman, R., & Sidman, M. (1967). *Neuroanatomy: a programmed text.* Boston: Little, Brown & Co.

Skinner, B. F. (1945). The operational analysis of psychological terms. *Psychological Review, 52,* 270–277.

Skinner, B. F. (1950). Are theories of learning necessary? *Psychological Review, 57,* 193–216.

Skinner, B. F. (1956). What is psychotic behavior? In F. Glide (Ed.), *Theory and treatment of the psychoses: some newer aspects.* St. Louis: Washington University Studies.

Skinner, B. F. (1957). *Verbal behavior.* New York: Appleton-Century-Crofts.

Skinner, B. F. (1958). Teaching machines. *Science, 128,* 969–977.

Skinner, B. F. (1966). An operant analysis of problem solving. In B. Kleinmuntz (Ed.), *Problem solving.* New York: John Wiley & Sons.

Skinner, B. F. (1969). *Contingencies of reinforcement: a theoretical analysis.* Englewood Cliffs, NJ: Prentice Hall.

Skinner, B. F. (1971). *Beyond freedom and dignity.* New York: Alfred A. Knopf.

Skinner, B. F. (1974). *About behaviorism.* New York: Knopf.

Skinner, B. F. (1977). The force of coincidence. *Humanist, 31*(3), 10–11.

Slavin, B. (1977, May 29). Hospital center for gambling addiction to open to Brooklyn, 2d in US. *New York Times,* pt. 1, p. 35, at 1–1.

Staddon, J. E. R. (1977). Schedule-induced behavior. In W. K. Honig and J. E. R. Staddon (Eds.), *Handbook of operant behavior.* Englewood Cliffs, NJ: Prentice-Hall.

Stent, G. S. (1976). The poverty of scientism and the promise of structuralist ethics. *Hastings Center Report,* (6), 32–40.

Swats, J. A. (Ed.) (1967). *Signal detection and recognition by human observers.* New York: John Wiley & Sons.

Szasz, T. S. (1961). *The myth of mental illness.* New York: Harper & Row.

Thompson. T., & Schuster. C. R. (1968). *Behavioral pharmacology.* Englewood Cliffs, NJ: Prentice-Hall.

Thorndike, E. L. (1913). *Educational psychology.* New York: Teachers College, Columbia University.

Ulrich, R. E., & Azrin, N. H. (1962). Reflexive fighting in response to aversive stimulation. *Journal of Experimental Analysis of Behavior, 5,* 511–520.

Valenstein, E. (1973). *Brain control: a critical examination of brain stimulation and psychosurgery.* New York: John Wiley & Sons.

Von Neumann. J., & Morgenstern, O. (1947). *Theory of games and economic behavior* (2nd ed.). Princeton: Princeton University Press.

Weiner, H. (1970). Human behavioral persistence. *Psychological Record, 20,* 445–456.

Weiss, B., & Laties. V. G. (Eds.) (1975). *Behavioral pharmacology: the current status.* Bethesda, MD: Federation of American Societies for Experimental Biology.

Wilson, E. O. (1975). *Sociobiology: the new synthesis.* Cambridge. MA: Harvard University.

Appendix A

The Search for an Effective Clinical Behavior Analysis: The Nonlinear Thinking of Israel Goldiamond*

T. V. Joe Layng

This paper has two purposes; the first is to reintroduce Goldiamond's constructional approach to clinical behavior analysis and to the field of behavior analysis as a whole, which, unfortunately, remains largely unaware of his nonlinear functional analysis and its implications. The approach is not simply a set of clinical techniques; instead it describes how basic, applied, and formal analyses may intersect to provide behavior-analytic solutions where the emphasis is on consequential selection. The paper takes the reader through a cumulative series of explorations, discoveries, and insights that hopefully brings the reader into contact with the power and comprehensiveness of Goldiamond's approach, and leads to an investigation of the original works cited. The second purpose is to provide the context of a life of scientific discovery that attempts to elucidate the variables and events that informed one of the most extraordinary scientific journeys in the history of behavior analysis, and expose the reader (especially young ones) to the exciting process of discovery followed by one of the field's most brilliant thinkers. One may perhaps consider this article a tribute to Goldiamond and his work, but the tribute is really to the process of scientific discovery over a professional lifetime.
Key words: Israel Goldiamond, nonlinear functional analysis, constructional approach

Israel Goldiamond must have become excited as he looked at his data. He and William Hawkins had just replicated results that had been obtained many times before. They had been very careful to follow the procedures precisely. The experimental subjects had been given a series of words made up of nonsense syllables to study. Some of the words were studied for a brief period of time, others for longer periods of time. Once studied, the stimuli were projected on a screen using a procedure known as the ascending method of limits. In this procedure stimuli are presented at increasing intensity or at slower speeds until a

* This work was originally published as Layng T. V. (2009). The search for an effective clinical behavior analysis: the nonlinear thinking of Israel Goldiamond. *The Behavior Analyst*, 32(1), 163–184. https://doi.org/10.1007/BF03392181

response matches the stimulus presented, as indicated by a score sheet. The investigators recorded each utterance of a word, and each score-sheet entry that corresponded to a stimulus presentation was scored as a correct identification. The score sheet was carefully constructed such that it contained the nonsense words carefully studied as well as those only briefly examined. Perception appeared to improve as a function of the training, producing what psychophysicists refer to as lower thresholds. The more the training a subject received, the more frequently the studied responses matched the score sheet, a complete replication. Almost everything was the same. The nonsense words studied were the same, the presentation method was the same, the speed of presentation was the same, and the score sheet used by the experimenter was the same. In fact, they had produced the familiar logarithmic function relating frequency of prior exposure to recognition threshold.

Goldiamond and Hawkins had made only one change to the procedure. No nonsense words had ever been presented. The subjects had been presented only smudges. The increasingly correct identifications that occurred as a function of training, as measured by matches to the experimenter's score sheet, had been obtained in the total absence of nonsense words. The result could not be attributed to perception, for there was nothing there to perceive.

THE FORMATIVE YEARS: GRADUATE WORK AT CHICAGO

Our story begins in the 1950s when Israel Goldiamond obtained a copy of Keller and Schoenfeld's (1950/ 1995) *Principles of Behavior*. It was his first in-depth introduction to what was then called operant psychology, and it would change his life. Goldiamond, a graduate student at the University of Chicago, had become keenly interested in perception and its study through what is called psychophysics. Psychophysics is one of the foundational areas of early experimental psychology. Great names in psychology such as Wundt, Fechner, Weber, and Stevens had led the way in building a behavioral science based on precise presentation of stimuli and equally precise measurement of human responses to those stimuli. Early on, it was referred to, often with a little hint of derogation, as "brass instrument psychology" because of the elaborate apparatus frequently required for work in the area.

Psychophysicists were carefully studying the relation between changes in stimuli and corresponding changes in behavior. The changes in behavior were taken to indicate changes in perception. The problem, however, was that the same stimuli appeared to be perceived differently as a function not only of a change in the stimulus but also of the way observers were asked to respond. One method of having an observer indicate whether or not a stimulus was seen frequently produced a different threshold from another method for exactly the same stimuli. A threshold was defined as a stimulus value, light intensity for example, at which 50% of the time an observer would say it was there and 50% of the time that it was not there. Often, unanticipated responses, considered errors by investigators, would occur. These errors required mathematical correction, specific to the procedure used, in order to get comparable results. For detailed reviews see Goldiamond (1958, 1962, 1964b) and Goldiamond and Thomas (1967/2004).

Further, two different response modalities, such as saying "yes" or "no" versus touching or not touching something, to indicate the presence or absence of a stimulus could produce differing results for the same stimulus presentations. At times, an observer would not report, or even emphatically deny, seeing a stimulus, but other behavior in some way indicated that the stimulus had been perceived. When this happened, unconscious, or what was called *subliminal*, perception was defined. That is, there was a difference between the spoken indicator response and some other, typically nonverbal, indicator response.

Investigators were also interested in the role of emotion, state of mind, or motivation in determining perception. Was an internal perceptual world changed that then determined how one responded to the external world? Many studies seemed to indicate that this may be the case. A range of variables, such as drives, needs, or even training, could influence this internal world. A hungry person might be able to smell food-related odors at lower thresholds than another who had just eaten; a sex offender might be able to detect sexually suggestive words more rapidly than typical individuals; a person who was trained on nonsense syllables might see them at lower thresholds than words that had not been so well learned. Research into hypnosis was suggesting that somehow the instructions of the hypnotist could radically alter the perceptual world of the observer. Instructed that red would always now be yellow, observers would say yellow when presented with red objects. Apparently, their color perception had changed. Psychophysical methods began to be applied to a range of behaviors, including the private world of the observer. For example, anxiety indexes based on psychophysical scaling methods were constructed; these methods showed promise and rapidly expanded into a separate field of mental and emotional testing.

What Goldiamond immediately realized from his reading of Keller and Schoenfeld (1950/1995) was that the responses used to indicate perception were, of course, operant behavior (i.e., behavior whose rate and form were functions of its consequences). As such, these indicator responses were subject to consequential control whether or not the investigator explicitly manipulated the consequences. Goldiamond reasoned that perhaps the difference in outcomes obtained when different indicator responses were used was a function of differences in personal consequential histories, both inside and outside the experimental context. In a series of innovative experiments, he and his colleagues were able to show that many of the differences in outcome occurred because the consequences of responding were simply being overlooked.

Over a period of years in the mid-1950s to the early 1960s, Goldiamond and his colleagues experimentally investigated many classes of perceptual behavior. They demonstrated that training did not alter the ability to perceive stimuli, but simply increased the frequency of those responses in comparison to other responses, thus resulting in more matches to the experimenter's score sheet (Goldiamond & Hawkins, 1958). For example, in the study that opened this article, greater training on certain nonsense words resulted in a greater tendency for the experimental subjects to say those words, thus making score-sheet matches more likely (the analysis applies equally well to the effects of food deprivation on smelling food-related odors, or the effects of sexual arousal on detecting sexually suggestive words; see Goldiamond, 1964b). They showed that hypnosis did not alter perception, but simply brought the indicator behavior under the control of the hypnotist's instructions (Goldiamond & Malpass, 1961). This was convincingly shown when experimental observers responded to the true afterimage of the real color presented and not to the afterimage of the instructed color. It was also demonstrated that implicit consequences could alter self-reports of internal states: College students who had never been in the military scored nearly identically to Korean War fighter pilots on surveys of emotional responses to combat when told to respond as a commanding officer might expect one to respond (Azrin, Holz, & Goldiamond, 1961). They also pointed out procedural difficulties that may occur in attempts to reinforce or punish conversational content (Azrin, Holz, Ulrich, & Goldiamond, 1961).

If the perception (i.e., indicator responses) of explicitly presented external stimuli could be shown to be a function of its consequences and related variables and not entirely of what was reported to be perceived, what about responses to one's own behavior? In a series of clever experiments, subjects attributed newly acquired stuttering to anxiety produced in a test situation, when in fact it was a function of a shock-avoidance schedule of which the subjects were entirely unaware (Flanagan, Goldiamond, & Azrin, 1959). What they were aware of were explanations of stuttering as caused by anxiety. Unaware of the consequences of their behavior, the reasons given by the subjects corresponded to the reasons that tended to be accepted by the audience, just as had the college students' responses to the survey, and who knows, perhaps even the pilots' (for a more comprehensive discussion of how these early studies may contribute to an understanding of causation and behavioral complexity, see Layng, 1995).

Another approach to perception was gaining popularity at about the same time. This approach, which Goldiamond helped to pioneer, became known as signal-detection theory (SDT). SDT provided methods for disentangling those variables that influence responding not related to the stimulus (response bias) from those that were a direct function of the stimulus (discriminability). In other words, SDT was able to separate the effects of the consequences of behavior from the ability of an observer to see (hear, smell, etc.) a stimulus. Here was an approach to perception that explicitly considered the effects of consequences on behavior and shared many of its procedures with those of operant psychology (see Goldiamond, 1964b; Goldiamond & Thompson, 1967/2004).

In one of the early experiments in this area, Goldiamond (1964b) was able to show that unconscious perception, that is, perception without awareness, was a function of differential consequences attached to two different indicator responses. Observers were seated in front of two lighted plastic panels; a faint triangle was presented on one of the two panels. After the triangle had been presented, the observers were instructed to press the panel with the triangle and say, "yes" if the triangle was there or "no" if it was not. The observers touched the panel on which the triangle was projected more often than they said "yes." Lower thresholds were obtained for panel presses than for "yes." The difference in thresholds obtained for the two different responses indicated the degree of unconscious perception that existed. Because the observers were more accurate when pressing than they were when saying "yes," their data indicated a subconscious perception of the triangle. That is, their spoken responses indicated that they did not see it, but their pressing responses indicated that they did. Goldiamond demonstrated that pressing a panel when a triangle was not there and saying "yes" when a triangle was not there may have different consequential histories, and that when procedures were put in place that reduced the effect of past consequences obtained outside the experiment for saying rather than doing, the thresholds converged. There was no subliminal perception (see also Goldiamond, 1958, 1959).

SDT also provided a basis for understanding the differences obtained using different psychophysical methods. It became evident that the probability of saying "yes" in the presence of the stimulus (a hit) was a function of the probability of saying "yes" in its absence (a false alarm). From the analysis of a 2 × 2 matrix, which has a minimum of two responses (yes and no) and a minimum of two states of the world (stimulus either absent or present), the effects of consequences and stimuli could be analyzed. By explicitly arranging consequences or payoffs, the likelihood of saying "yes" when the target stimulus was present and "no" when it was absent could be systematically controlled. When the payoff for saying "yes" with the target stimulus absent was manipulated, the frequency of saying "yes" with the target stimulus present would also change. This was observed even though the consequences for saying "yes" with the target stimulus present remained unchanged. Even as the false-alarm rate varies and the hit rate correspondingly covaries, the underlying discriminability of the stimulus remains unchanged. When one sees a low false-alarm rate, one also sees a low hit rate; a high false-alarm rate results in a high hit rate. That is, the ratio of false alarms to hits remains mostly unchanged as the consequences are changed for a given range of stimulus presentations.

SDT allowed the separate evaluation of two key aspects of perception, discriminability and response bias. *Discriminability* was defined by how discrepant the target stimulus was from other stimuli. *Response bias* was defined as a preference for saying "yes" or "no." Discriminability combined with response bias to determine the overall likelihood of saying "yes." Here was the answer to why there were differences in results given the different psycho-physical procedures used for nearly a century. Each procedure engendered a slightly different response bias. SDT now allowed the separate evaluation of the contribution of each to an observer's overall score. False positives and false negatives were not errors, but instead were the logical and sensible outcome of their consequences (Goldiamond, 1964b; Goldiamond & Thompson, 1967/2004).

Experiments showed that the more ambiguous the situation, the more an observer's behavior was a function of its consequences (reflected as response bias) and less a function of the presence or absence of the stimulus. The important discovery that the probability of saying "yes" in the presence of a target stimulus was a function not only of its consequences but also of the consequences for saying "yes" in its absence was not overlooked by Goldiamond. He clearly saw that to fully understand complex behavior, one had to consider entire sets, or matrices, of contingencies, rather than focus on just one.

If reports of public events were so governed, then reports of private or inner events had to be similarly governed. And because, by their nature, private events were necessarily ambiguous, publicly speaking about those events was even more likely to be governed by their consequences. Goldiamond found that what people said about themselves, and the world around them, was not merely a function of past consequences for similar responses in those situations but was also a function of past consequences for saying something different on similar occasions.

It became clear that much of verbal behavior, particularly in ambiguous situations, was largely a function of its consequences and other related variables, and that the pure discrimination was indeed rare. Further, it was not enough to look at or arrange consequences for a target response; attention had to be paid to alternative responses as well. Speech content as well as other behaviors were more likely to be guided by these alternative relations than not (Goldiamond, 1958, 1962, 1964b). This early work helped to provide the foundation for the search for a comprehensive behavior analysis that would continue the rest of Goldiamond's life.

EMERGING CLINICAL INSIGHTS

While a graduate student at Chicago, Goldiamond had taken a course from the famous clinical psychologist Carl Rogers. Although he was not inspired by Rogers' approach, he became interested in how a consequential analysis could inform therapeutic practice. After graduation, Goldiamond began a two-pronged career, one that continued his pursuit of an experimental analysis of behavior, both human and animal, and also one that focused on behavior of clinical importance. The two interests often intersected and were treated with equal rigor.

Over the next few years, from the late 1950s to the late 1960s, while Goldiamond was at Southern Illinois University, Arizona State University, the Institute for Behavioral Research, and Johns Hopkins University, procedures were developed to analyze, understand, and intervene in behavior, often verbal, of clinical interest. Speech was reinstated in mute psychotics (Issacs, Thomas, & Goldiamond, 1960), stuttering was analyzed and treatment procedures were designed (Flanagan, Goldiamond, & Azrin, 1958, 1959; Goldiamond, 1965b; Goldiamond, Atkinson, & Bilger, 1962; Goldiamond & Flanagan, 1959; continuous research and development would yield a systematic program that eventually taught over 200 stutterers to speak fluently), methods of self-control were developed (Goldiamond, 1965a), psychotic hallucinations were analyzed in the context of psychophysical research (Goldiamond,

1964b), a behavioral approach to moral behavior was described (Goldiamond, 1968), and a functional analysis of the content of speech in therapeutic sessions was undertaken, as well as how behavioral interactions within a therapeutic session could result in changes outside the session (Goldiamond & Dyrud, 1968; Goldiamond, Dyrud, & Miller, 1965).

Together with colleagues such as Nate Azrin, behavioral psychoanalyst Jarl Dyrud, and many others, Goldiamond began to develop insights as to what constitutes an effective functional analytic approach to psychotherapy. Goldiamond and Azrin had a profound influence on one another. In giving his eulogy at Goldiamond's memorial service, Azrin described Goldiamond's influence on everything from the token economy to his own approach to marital therapy. Goldiamond would likely have had similar things to say about Azrin. Other work in the operant laboratory helped to elucidate variables that would be of considerable importance for clinical analysis and treatment.

Goldiamond often drew on these insights for his work with patients. Two in particular drew his attention. In 1960, Murray Sidman had published some of his observations about some possible normal sources of pathological behavior in an article published in *Science* (see also Sidman, 1958). Given certain arrangements, monkeys would apparently work to receive shocks. In a series of brilliantly designed experiments, Sidman demonstrated the important role of behavioral history and the interaction of concurrent consequential contingencies in understanding and making sense of seemingly paradoxical behavior. Estes and Skinner (1941) had shown that the presentation of a clicker paired with shock could suppress lever pressing on some interval schedules, but if a monkey had a history of pressing a lever to avoid shocks, the opposite happened; the pressing was instead facilitated. Further, shock could be made contingent on lever pressing after the avoidance schedule had been terminated, and lever pressing would actually increase, producing more shocks. All the animal had to do was stop pressing and no shocks would be delivered. It was, in essence, trapped by its history of available alternatives. This was not psychopathology, but a sensible outcome of actions taken in the past to reduce shock frequency.

Sidman (1960) also showed how patterns maintained by two different consequences, in this case pressing a lever to avoid shock and pulling a chain to produce food, could become intertwined. He reasoned that if the two operants were indeed a function of their separate histories, discontinuing the shock-avoidance schedule and introducing unavoidable shocks should result in an increase in lever pressing and a decrease in chain pulling, in accord with his and Estes and Skinner's (1941) results. It did not turn out that way. Both responses' frequencies increased. One conventional interpretation was that the increases were a function of the underlying emotional response to the shock, a common pathological perspective. Sidman instead showed that the result was a function of an adventitious arrangement of the consequential contingencies and a sensible outcome of that arrangement. When schedules were changed such that the effects of lever pressing were clearly separated from the effects of chain pulling, the results were as predicted earlier. The important lesson inherent in these studies was that the consequential history of the behavior under investigation was critical to understanding current patterns, and that seemingly pathological behavior could occur as a function of quite sensible responding to quite prosaic behavioral processes. Further, simply considering the apparently pathological pattern, without reference to its alternatives and their consequential histories, would yield an incomplete picture at best, and result in a completely wrong analysis at worst.

Another set of experiments that further supported Goldiamond's emerging approach was a series of studies performed by Holz and Azrin (1961) showing that punishment could be a discriminative stimulus for reinforcement. From time to time, pecks to a disk mounted on a wall provided food to a hungry pigeon, but did so only if an electric shock followed each peck. Unshocked pecks to the disk did not result in food. The pigeons quickly learned that no shock meant no food, and that shock meant food. If they pecked and there was no shock, they would stop pecking, but if a shock were provided they would peck. The presence of electric shock occasioned the very behavior that produced it. If one were to only observe those pecks that produced shock and overlooked those that resulted in food, one might consider the pecking to be an indicator of psychopathology.

But why peck at all? The answer from the pigeons' point of view was unambiguous: peck, get shocked, eventually get fed; do something else, don't get shocked, starve. When one considered the alternatives available to the pigeon, the pecking for shock made absolute sense. Further, Goldiamond reasoned, one could arrange conditions in which pigeons would work to turn on the shock if it were absent. The pain of one's actions may be necessary to achieve an ultimate payoff. And, when available alternatives are considered, that pain, and the pursuit of those conditions or life contexts that result in such pain, may not be maladaptive at all. In fact, it may be considered quite adaptive and sensible. The therapeutic approach suggested here was to find or construct an alternative that could provide the same payoff, but without the pain.

THE EXTENSION OF A FUNCTIONAL BEHAVIOR ANALYSIS TO CLINICAL TREATMENT

The promise of the rapidly growing operant literature, together with his own previous work, made Goldiamond's collaboration with the physician and psychoanalyst Jarl Dyrud an exciting opportunity to test the power of a functional analysis of behavior in the clinic. They began their collaboration in the mid-1960s while Goldiamond was executive director of the Institute for Behavioral Research. Goldiamond would sit in on Dyrud's therapy sessions taking notes, providing a contingency analysis of what transpired, and making suggestions. The two would remain lifelong friends.

Dyrud quickly came to see the power of the analysis Goldiamond provided. Some years later, Dyrud (1971) suggested that psychoanalysts should embrace behavioral functional analysis as the tool that they had been seeking all of these years in their effort to understand the unconscious. He wrote, "Our assumption is that seemingly erratic behavior is in fact consequential, often at a level below awareness, and that the elucidation of its consequences is our major vehicle for treatment (making the unconscious conscious)" (p. 302). In 1968, their collaboration resulted in a paper titled, "Some Applications and Implications of Behavioral Analysis for Psychotherapy." It, along with an earlier article (Goldiamond et al., 1965), were perhaps the first papers on the use of a consequential functional analysis for adult psychotherapy. This was not systematic desensitization, or token economies, or the direct reinforcement of verbal content, or the use of rewards and punishment to get someone to behave in ways the patient or therapist thought was good for them. Instead, it was the direct use of an explicit functional analysis to help individuals change their context for living, that is, their contingencies.

The Goldiamond and Dyrud collaboration also produced some very interesting clinical experiments; one in particular deserves elaboration. They placed a psychiatrist in one room and a patient in another. A type of one-way mirror separated the rooms such that the patient could see the psychiatrist as long as a light was directly shining on the therapist. They then linked the brightness of the light to speech rate. If the patient maintained a specified rate of speaking, the therapist remained visible; if the rate dropped off, the room would darken, making the therapist difficult to see. This relation was never described to the patient. By manipulating speech rate, they could change both affect and conversation content. High rate requirements produced statements of anger, frustration, and anxiety that the patient would attribute to his life situation; even higher rates could produce psychotic-like responding, with near delusional behavior, "word salad"-like responses, and often agitated roaming around the room. Access to the psychotherapist was a powerful reinforcer. It is doubtful that this experiment could be conducted today.[1]

It became clear to Goldiamond that clinically relevant behavior, including verbal content and affect, were all adaptively a function of consequential selection. It was also clear that consequences came in packages that contained both costs and benefits. Keeping the psychiatrist visible was a potent explicit reinforcer; however, it came at a cost of finding things of clinical relevance to say, an implicit requirement of continued therapy. Extrapolating from his experience with SDT and work performed in the operant laboratory, Goldiamond surmised that these consequence packages had to be considered not only for the "symptom" but also for available alternative patterns. Goldiamond saw that once one examined both the relative costs and benefits for what he would later call the disturbing pattern and those for alternative patterns available to the patient, the function of the behavior was revealed; more than that, why the individual behaved as he or she did became clear.

STIMULUS CLASSES AND ABSTRACTIONAL, INSTRUCTIONAL, AND DIMENSIONAL CONTROL IN THE CLINIC

Goldiamond continued to publish on perception and how various stimuli interacted with behavior as a function of certain consequences. In 1962, he described how both stimulus and response classes could be formed and how these classes may be extended to include other stimuli or responses, and how, "once a class is established, contingencies applied to one member of a class tend to affect other members of the class" (p. 303).

In 1966 Goldiamond elaborated on the important distinction between dimensional and abstractional or instructional control, and how each could be transferred separately or together. To somewhat over simplify, dimensional control was *what* one responded to and abstractional control was *how* one responded to it. For instance, one may respond to an airplane by stating its color, its weight, the number of passengers carried, or a variety of other features. Responding to the plane (vs. something else) indicates dimensional control, and responding along any of a multitude of features represents abstractional control. One can transfer abstractional or relational responding across different stimuli that vary greatly in appearance. For example, color naming can be transferred from naming the color of an airplane to naming the color of a house. One can establish abstractional control by comparison (e.g., larger than); it can also be established through a common response (e.g., stopping at a railroad crossing, a stoplight, etc.) or by various forms of stimulus pairing. Both dimensional control and abstractional control can be transferred independently or together, as Goldiamond (1964a, 1966) demonstrated with a program that precisely sequenced a series of letters and words. As a result of the sequencing, observers who begin the sequence classifying letter groups or words by the presence of the letter B are led instead to classify by the presence of words that reflect male gender (and reject those words containing B if they do not reflect male gender), without hearing a verbal description of either relation. (During this period, Goldiamond & Thompson [1967/2004] produced one half of a planned wide-ranging book on behavior analysis that included the most systematic treatment of stimulus control ever written.)

Goldiamond and Dyrud (1968) went on to postulate that some forms of the psychoanalytic concept of transference might have a basis in such relations. Talking about how interacting with one's wife is similar to how one interacted with one's mother may be an example of such control. But there was a twist. Such comparisons did not necessarily reveal that the relationship with the mother, or what happened in that relationship, was necessarily causally linked, but that, of all the thousands of interactions that had occurred, the patient had chosen this one to describe. A similar analysis could be made of remembered dreams. Both past interactions and recent dreams may speak to current contingencies. Each may help to elucidate current abstractional control and the consequences that maintain it.

Often, encouraging a change in abstractional control in a therapeutic session, that is, establishing a different way of responding to an event, could be transferred to events outside the session. They noted that the effectiveness of such transfer frequently depended on how patients responded to therapist-supplied stimuli and, in turn, how the therapist responds to the apparent abstractional control as it occurs. The therapist responds to the theme and not necessarily the precise words chosen by the patient. Accordingly, the role of metaphor in facilitating not only analysis but also transfer was described in the 1968 article and expanded on in later work in the 1970s. (See, e.g., Goldiamond, 1974a, 1975a. Two of Goldiamond's students, Layng & Andronis, 1984, later published an article that extensively discussed the use of metaphor interpretation in the treatment of delusions and hallucinations.)

Goldiamond and Dyrud (1968) considered potentiating variables, or what are now often called motivative or establishing operations, as critical to successful outcomes. They argued that understanding the sources of consequence potentiation is critical to successful therapy, and further, that yet other elements of the psychoanalytic concept of transference may be analyzed, in part, through a consideration of potentiation. Equally important was the potentiation of reinforcers that could maintain patient behavior within a session: "What may be a critical reinforcer in psychotherapy is change in referent behaviors outside. Events in the session that are related to such change may thereby become linked to them as reinforcers themselves" (p. 74).

As further work would continue to show (Goldiamond, 1969), the key to extension, and to meaningful change outside the therapeutic session, is how events in the session affect the consequential relations that maintain the disturbing patterns outside the session. Although it may be the case that "once a class is established, contingencies applied to one member of a class tend to affect other members of the class," as noted earlier such change is maintained only if it is supported by a change in the referent consequential contingencies.

THE RETURN TO CHICAGO: THE CONSTRUCTIONAL APPROACH AND NONLINEAR VERSUS LINEAR ANALYSIS

In 1968, Goldiamond accepted a position as professor in the Departments of Behavioral Sciences (Biopsychology), Psychiatry, Medicine and in the College (the undergraduate school) at the University of Chicago; Dyrud accepted an appointment in the Department of Psychiatry and ultimately became chair for a time while at Chicago. Years of clinical research, including a rigorous research program conducted at the Behavior Analysis Research Laboratory of the Department of Psychiatry ultimately led to the publication of what Goldiamond (1974b) called a "constructional approach." This was groundbreaking work, a functional analysis that considered the consequences and related variables not only of disturbing patterns but of their alternatives as well. Rather than simply considering a linear occasion behavior-consequence sequence, this was a nonlinear approach in which the behavior being investigated was understood to be a function of multiple intersecting contingencies.[2]

When investigators considered only the consequences for the disturbing behavior, it often seemed as though the disturbing pattern made no sense and must be a function of some type of internal emotional or cognitive state. However, an examination of the available alternative consequential contingencies, reminiscent of the payoff matrix of SDT, quickly dispelled this notion.[3] Further, Goldiamond and his students found that changes in reported emotions and cognitions tracked changes in the contingency matrix. Emotions and cognitions lost their causal status once the entire matrix was described. They did, however, remain an important source of information in helping to identify those relations of which the emotions themselves were also a function.

Goldiamond quickly came to understand that the goal of therapy was not to directly control, change, or suppress emotions or cognition, but instead to sensitize the patient to them, use them as indicators of the relevant consequential contingencies, and to build on their current repertoires so as to arrange new contingencies. Patients were taught that their disturbing patterns were quite sensible and often nearly heroic responses to the contingency matrix in which they found themselves, and that their behavior was neither maladaptive nor pathological. The approach is illustrated by an example provided by Goldiamond (1975b) about a woman with a debilitating phobia that often left her confined to her bed:

> She was immobilized thereby and her husband swept and cleaned the house every morning (to clear it of vermin), brought her breakfast in bed, and washed the dishes (to deter vermin) before leaving for work. Whenever she recovered somewhat, his attentiveness waned. The phobia was costly: she could not resume the professional work she had enjoyed, nor could they go out together at night; further her in-laws were suggesting divorce. The benefits to recovery are obvious, as is the matrix. There is a metaphor involved. Labeling the disturbing behavior as a psychiatric problem is essential to the matrix. The patient would not get the accruing benefits if she simply told her husband: "Look, you've been putting work ahead of me and everything else since we've been married. I've worked to keep this marriage together. How about you?" Indeed, earlier efforts in this direction had been extinguished. Numerous psychiatric problems have this legitimate labeling function. Labeling theorists who denounce such terms might reflect further on this metaphorical use for the patient, rather than upon the psychiatrist's benefits and the crippling effects of the label upon the patient. It is the contingency matrix that produces the disturbing effects and governs the behavior and the experienced emotions or thought patterns. (p. 43)

THE ROLE OF EMOTION IN CLINICAL BEHAVIOR ANALYSIS

Emotion theorists had for some time argued about the role of emotions. Some argued that emotions could cause behavior. One is afraid, therefore, one flees; the fleeing may reduce the fear and thus reward running. Others argued that, no, one runs away from something and feels fear as a result of running, the behavior of running away causes the feeling of fear. Goldiamond saw from what was now years of work in the clinic and laboratory that neither explanation was adequate. Instead, he found that both fleeing and feeling fear were a function of the consequential contingencies; one did not cause the other. This was an important discovery. One does not run from the bear because one is afraid, and one is not afraid because one is running from the bear—one is both running and afraid because there is a bear close on one's heels. Fear describes a specific functional relation between behavior and its consequences. It describes the situation in which one's behavior is reinforced by putting distance between oneself and some other thing or event. Anger, which so often goes hand in hand with fear, describes those conditions in which one's behavior is reinforced by creating distance between oneself and an event by removing or driving off the event. Emotions, therefore, may be considered as describing or amplifying specific contingency relations, and specific contingencies can be described by specific emotions (Goldiamond, 1974b, 1975b, 1979b; Layng, 2006).[4]

The implications were stunning. It was becoming evident that our emotions evolved to aid us in navigating complex contingencies that are a part of a complex social world. We are oblivious to most of the contingencies that govern our day-to-day behavior. Nonetheless, it is important that we come in contact with them and act accordingly; we do this through our emotions. Clinically, emotions could be used to uncover those contingencies, to make the unconscious conscious, by making the implicit consequential contingencies explicit.

THE PATIENT AS COINVESTIGATOR IN ANALYZING NONLINEAR RELATIONS AND PLANNING TOPICAL AND SYSTEMIC TREATMENT

But how was this discovered? As part of the research protocol, patients were asked to keep records. These records, some of which were published in the appendix of Goldiamond (1974b), were filled out by the patient on a daily basis between visits. Understanding that record keeping and what was recorded are operant behaviors, it was important to make sure these records formed the basis of patient–therapist interactions. A great deal of time was devoted to examining and analyzing the daily logs in each session (see Goldiamond & Schwartz, 1975). If a log was brought to a session not filled out, session time was used to retroactively fill in the missing times. This joint evaluation led to many discoveries that might not otherwise have been made. For example, it was noticed that events on one day could potentiate reinforcers for different behaviors on another day. For instance, on some days phobic behavior may have no discernible consequence; however, at other times, the consequences, which ranged from control over the behavior of a spouse to avoiding an unpleasant task, were easily identified. It became apparent that if the phobic response occurred only on the occasions in which it obviously paid off, it would cease to work on those occasions. To potentiate the social consequences for the phobic response on one occasion, the behavior had to occur on other occasions in which there were no discernible social consequences or even when a cost might be observed. Just as shock had become discriminative for food in the Holz and Azrin (1961) experiments, the cost of the phobia may have to be evident if others are to provide the consequences that maintain phobic or other disturbing behavior. Chance (1994) fittingly called this Goldiamond's paradox (see also Layng & Andronis, 1984).

Records were not, however, simply indicators of disturbing patterns, but were used to find when things went right and why. Emphasis was placed on what was going on when the patient felt good, and how this was achieved. Each week there were goals to be achieved based on the previous week's successes. Setbacks were treated as expected outcomes of any worthwhile effort, and were occasions for further contingency analysis.

When the social consequences were no longer potent or when the best interests of the patient were served by giving up the symptom, it was easily understood why the patient was now seeking therapy. Patients' logs frequently showed that the disturbing pattern involved costs for others as well as for the patient. Those close to the patient might not easily accept an immediate dropping of the symptom. Also, it might be necessary to build certain skills for situations avoided in the past. When a phobia was involved, a simple intervention might involve understanding that the phobic feelings were likely to have occurred in situations in which there was no direct payoff, and to use those feelings as indicators to stop and examine the situation and see what one could do that, step by step, would lead to coming into contact with new experiences and new consequences. The phobic feelings were to be treated as a natural outcome of the individual's personal history. For many, this was all that was required. If, say, spousal involvement was the critical consequence, and available alternative patterns in the patient's repertoire had not been successful in obtaining such involvement, "topical" interventions, directed exclusively at the presenting complaint (e.g., fear of cockroaches) are likely to be only minimally successful. These include working on the fear responses directly or on the avoidance of fearful emotions. Intervention has to be directed elsewhere. The relationship with the spouse must be the focus. As the relationship changes, and the consequences that maintain the phobia (spousal involvement) are either obtained elsewhere or are no longer potent, the phobic symptoms may simply drop out of the repertoire, or the change may allow a topical intervention to replace the phobia with other less troublesome patterns.

A range of specialty logs was developed, including social interaction logs, emotional responding logs, and others as required for a particular life situation. One's thoughts and personal observations were regularly included. Often, the records indicated incidents of application, or self-control, of what had been learned from the logs. From Goldiamond (1976a):

> I shall cite the report of an out-patient upon his return from vacation. He had had a history of hospitalization for schizophrenia and his brother was recently hospitalized for the same problem. During his vacation his wife walked out on him, leaving him alone in the motel. "I found myself sitting in bed the whole morning, and staring at my rigid finger," he said. "So I asked myself: 'Now what would Dr. Goldiamond say was the reason I was doing this?' He'd ask what consequences would ensue. And I'd say: 'Hospitalization.' And he'd say: "That's right! Just keep it up and they'll take you away.' And then he'd say: 'But what would you be getting there that you're not getting now?' And I'd say: 'I'll be taken care of.' And he'd say: 'You're on target. But is there some way you can get this consequence without going to the hospital and having another hospitalization on your record?' And then I'd think a while and say: 'Hey! My sister. She's a motherly type, and she lives a hundred miles away.'" He reported that he dragged himself together, packed, and hitch-hiked to his sister who took him in with open arms. The education occurred in the process of the analysis of several months of written records. (p. 33)

Increasingly, effective treatment required that for many symptoms, patterns other than the presenting complaint (the original symptoms) needed to be considered. Once these other patterns and their consequences were addressed, the symptom often dropped out with no need to attend directly to the disturbing pattern. This type of intervention would come to be called *systemic*, as distinguished from *topical*. Topical interventions directly address the presenting complaint. Both types of intervention may employ a nonlinear functional analysis and are not necessarily mutually exclusive (Goldiamond, 1979b,1984; Layng & Andronis, 1984). For example, patients who engage in certain forms of obsessive compulsive behavior benefited from combining certain topical interventions similar to those found in habit reversal procedures (Azrin & Nunn, 1973) with a systemic intervention targeted toward building repertoires, the absence of which was the obsessive compulsive disorder.

THE IMPORTANCE OF VERBAL BEHAVIOR

Goldiamond's work with, and understanding of, verbal behavior was also important to the success of the approach. An interview strategy was developed that, with amazing regularity, often indicated the important nonlinear consequence relations that were maintaining the disturbing pattern. By focusing on outcomes to be achieved, rather than on deficits to be eliminated, contingencies were uncovered and new ones built that resulted in patients coming to control their own lives and plans for the future. Analysis and planning continue well after the initial interview. A poignant example was provided by Goldiamond (1974b):

> Can one deliver reinforcement to behaviors such as hallucinations that are almost universally regarded as pathological? Indeed, they enter into the diagnosis of schizophrenia. The parents of a woman of 22, so classified, reported that she was hallucinating a husband and children at the dinner table and engaging them in extended conversation. If they ignored her (extinction),

they knew she would escalate (e.g., hallucinate pregnancy, etc.) until they were forced to reply. If they were punitive, she might start screaming or might stay away from the table and undo their intense efforts to get her there. If they agreed or inquired after the "family" (reinforcement) this, too, might escalate the pattern. The tactics recommended were based on the following rationale. A child's report card has A's, C's and F's. The parents can complain about the failing grades, cite the A's to indicate she can do better, or simply praise heavily for the A's. The hallucinatory patterns were to be regarded in the same way: what is there about them that can be reinforced? Most 22-year-old women are married, and neighboring daughters were no exception. Her mother said, next time: "Sally, you don't know how delighted I am to hear you considering marriage just like — and —. Believe me, nothing would make father and me happier than," etc., "and that's why we're doing — and —, to make that day come sooner." The parents had to be as ingenious as their daughter in changing the words as they retained the theme to keep up with her changing presentations of the same theme (she had had considerably more experience). By the third week, hallucinations were replaced by conversations with the existent family. What the parents said was true, and she was treated with responses that respected her dignity and also moved the program along. (pp. 51–52; see also Layng & Andronis, 1984, for additional examples)

Informed by years of research on instructional and abstractional control, Goldiamond wrote extensively on the topic of rules and their role in understanding behavior. He was quick to point out that any consequentially governed behavior could be described as meeting contingency rules for reinforcement. That is, once criteria required for reinforcement were identified, one could describe the rule for reinforcement availability. This rule could then be provided to others, and the behavior that ensued would be maintained as long as the behavior continued to provide potent consequences within its contingency context (Goldiamond, 1966; Goldiamond & Thompson, 1967/ 2004). Skinner (1966) alluded to this when he wrote of the "inspection of reinforcement contingencies." Goldiamond, however, cautioned that patterns, which may be overlooked by either patients or therapists, other than the ones established by the rule might provide more benefits with fewer costs. Regardless, Goldiamond (1978/1983) maintained that rule statement was irrelevant to contingency control, and that the statement of a rule by the patient or therapist was no guarantee that the contingencies were accurately being described. Rules do not cause behavior, nor does behavior cause rules or insight into them:

In situations outside the laboratory, people often follow rules of conduct relatable to histories of Oc-(BR→S) relations; they may then (or may not) explicitly state the induced rules to others and to themselves. ... Thus, as used here, awareness, insight, and explicit induction of rules are not the epiphenomena to which operationism often assigns them. They do not linearly cause behavior (OcR→Awareness [etc.] R→ Behavior), nor do behaviors cause awareness, etc. (OcR→BehaviorR→Awareness). Both awareness (insight, explicit induction) and behavior are governed by the contingencies and their histories. The fact that one can occasionally precede the other indicates causality no more than it does in emotion and behavior. And, as in different classes of behavior with different histories, they should not be expected to have identical contingency relations. ... If presence of insight, or awareness of contingencies, is irrelevant to control by contingencies, instructions on the nature of the present contingencies or of those to be instituted may facilitate occurrence of the required patterns, or may not, depending on the conditions. Among the critical conditions is whether or not consequences follow upon behavior in accord with instructions about the rule. (p. 14)

He noticed that patients might state rules for their patterns, or therapists might describe patient patterns in terms of rules or "misrules." It became obvious, however, that the rule stating and the patterns observed are both governed by alternative sets of consequential arrangements. That is, each may have its own consequences and alternatives. He noted a further caution: Rules may be abstracted from adventitious relations, where from time to time consequences may occur but may not be functionally related to the behavior. He admonished both patients and therapists to be cautious when stating rules that describe apparent consequential relations (Goldiamond, 1978/1983):

> Presentation of statements of contingencies may be used to induce rules which may then function instructionally. In any case of instruction-governed behavior, if the contingency rule applied is incongruent with the actual Oc-(BR→S) arrangements, instructional control may be transient. However, precaution is necessary here. Adventitiously reinforced behavior is likely to be reinforced only intermittently. Related abstractions and instructions induced from these are, because of the adventitious reinforcement attached to behavior under their control, likely to be spurious. Because of the intermittency of the reinforcement, the spurious instructions are likely to be long-lived (cf. Skinner, 1977), despite the simultaneous availability of less spurious instructional and abstractional systems. (p. 15)

For the patient, this means that the putative controlling consequences observed may not be maintaining the disturbing patterns or may be maintaining them only adventitiously. As a result, alternatives may be available that either had been overlooked by the patient, or in the past have been unavailable, or might become available with a relatively small change in repertoire. A therapist might be tempted to suggest a patient may be following a defective rule or is insensitive to his or her consequential contingencies. As noted earlier, another approach is to consider the behavior to be the sensible outcome of a consequential history not unlike that described by Sidman (1960). It is a combination of that history and current consequences within the contingency matrix that accounts for the pattern. Often, the alternative contingencies as experienced by the patient, and what Goldiamond called "developmental costs" (i.e., the effort involved in learning or transferring repertoires), may keep patients boxed in to their particular contingency matrix.

Other relations were noted as well. Disturbing patterns that apparently produced no consequences other than aversive ones were often found to be the lesser of two or more evils when available alternative relations were considered. The patterns appeared irrational or maladaptive only in a linear "lone contingency" framework. Overlooking the fact that a pattern can produce more than one consequence and thereby considering only the costs and ignoring the benefits, especially in terms of the available alternatives, was another outcome of a linear analysis. In addition, there was the recognition of "vestigial" patterns. These are patterns that at one time paid off but do so no longer, or are now maintained by sporadic adventitious consequences. These patterns are largely maintained by the cost of giving them up, as noted above.

No single rule, approach, procedure, or diagnostically based intervention is possible. Matching treatment to diagnostic topography may have limited success, except perhaps when the presenting complaint is a vestigial pattern, or when there has been a change in the contingency matrix prior to seeking therapy. Each individual's multiple contingency context, and the histories of those contingency relations, need to be examined. This is why Goldiamond (1974b) required his students to begin their case presentations like this:

A. Introduction
   1. Identifying information
      Brief description of patient and a few qualifying statements which are relevant to what follows.
   2. Background for the program

Use A3 as the resolution toward which this presentation is directed. Weave in various items from questionnaire and other sources to present a coherent picture of a person functioning highly competently, given his circumstances and implicit or explicit goals. Present the history of the person as an example of such competence, giving evidence wherever available.

3. Symptom as costly operant

Infer how, as a result of A2, the patterns shaped and reinforced up to now are now too costly or otherwise jeopardizing the patient. Infer what reinforcers are presently maintaining patterns, sources, and type of jeopardy and its source. This should be brief and simply stated as what led up to this. (p. 80; for the rest of the case presentation guide, see Goldiamond, 1974b)

The therapeutic process always began by asking patients what it would be like for them 6 months after liberation day from their problems. Within the first few sessions, observable goals were described that both therapist and patient agreed to work to achieve. Sometimes these goals would change, but if so, they would be clearly stated in terms of observable outcomes. If a person came into therapy because of panic attacks, it would be ascertained what the individual would be doing if the attacks were gone. The goal would not be to eliminate the attacks, but to produce the outcomes achievable only if the attacks were gone. This was contrasted with the individual's current situation. Patient strengths and past successes were also investigated. This was the starting point for the program. An initial contingency analysis of the disturbing pattern and its alternatives was made from data obtained from the original interview and patient logs (and, at times, speaking with others). This analysis was presented to the patient; no records, notes, or other write-ups were kept from the individual seeking help. Every week subgoals based on the past week's successes and related to the program goals were identified and methods suggested, derived from the ongoing contingency analysis, for reaching them. As described above, patient records in the form of the logs documented the application of the procedures, provided occasions for analysis, and showed what was successful and what was not. Success was defined by whether or not the patient achieved the stated observable outcomes (for a more detailed discussion of the processes, see Goldiamond, 1974b, 1975b, 1979b, 1984; Goldiamond& Schwartz, 1975; Layng, 2006; Merley & Layng, 1976).[5]

EXTENSION AND APPLICATION: TOPICAL AND SYSTEMIC INTERVENTIONS

As the decade of the 1970s came to a close, research efforts were increasingly directed toward understanding the topical versus systemic intervention differences. Travis (1982) investigated what would happen if patients whose initial analysis indicated a topical intervention was sufficient were placed in a systemic intervention, and those whose initial analysis indicated a systemic intervention was necessary were placed in a topical only intervention. The data were informative: As predicted, progress in therapy appeared to be contingent on the proper intervention.

The logs also pointed to another key distinction. This time it was the difference between emotions as contingency descriptors and emotional behavior. For instance, acting angrily or depressively might not always reflect contingencies that describe anger or feeling depressed. If a contingency that produced an emotion also produced related behavior, it could be selected by its consequences just like any other operant. If feeling angry and having the physiological indicators often associated with reports of such feeling were required to meet the consequential requirements, then they would occur. It became clear that physiological or organic responses could enter into the definition of the operant. This was highlighted when a case of stigmata (bleeding from the palms) was shown to be an operant and was successfully treated systemically by addressing marital relations, and when intense and uncontrollable blushing was successfully treated with a topical functional analysis (Goldiamond, 1974b). In the systemic case, marital issues needed attention; the stigmata themselves were not directly addressed. In the topical case, the patient was taught not to try to fight or control her blushing, but instead to heed it and use the early sensations as an indicator that she needed to intervene in a social situation that might lead to intense blushing. Special procedures were developed that helped to distinguish between emotions as contingency descriptors or amplifiers and emotional behavior as operants or, as in the case of blushing just cited, some of each (for a more recent and extensive discussion, see Layng, 2006).

Goldiamond (1975a) published a paper that formally described his nonlinear or alternative sets approach and its implications for behavioral formulations in general. Later (1976b) he gave an inside look at his personal use of this approach by describing its application to his own injury that left him in a wheelchair (see also Goldiamond, 1974a). He extended his nonlinear analysis to problems of social significance (1974b), and continued to do so through a series of publications that directly addressed those issues (Goldiamond, 1975c, 1976b, 1977). In 1978, Goldiamond's Midwestern Association of Behavior Analysis (which later became the Association for Behavior Analysis) presidential address formally provided a "Programming Contingency Analysis of Mental Health" (Goldiamond, 1978/1983). It was brilliant, and detailed a comprehensive behavior-analytic approach to understanding clinically relevant behavior, including the relations among behavior, genetics, and other physiological variables. He later submitted a revised and expanded version as a book chapter that was to be a part of a larger compilation, only later to withdraw it when the editors asked that it be shortened. Copies do exist of this work, and may yet be published. Goldiamond (1979a) first publicly described in print his discovery of the distinction between topical and systemic interventions.

Over the next several years, Goldiamond and his students would continue to refine and extend the nonlinear analysis, both in the clinic and in the laboratory. Schedules of reinforcement were shown to influence gastrointestinal behavior when schedule-induced defecation was discovered (Gimenez, Andronis, & Goldiamond, 1987; Rayfield, Segal, & Goldiamond, 1982). The implications for the treatment of irritable bowel syndrome and similar conditions were investigated in conjunction with physicians from the department of medicine. Changes in reinforcement schedules for key pecking were shown to result in the recurrence of extinguished head banging in pigeons, which replicated similar observations made in the clinic and suggested that relapse was a normal rather than pathological behavioral process (Layng, Andronis, & Goldiamond, 1999). Pigeon research showed how component repertoires that were a function of one set of consequences could combine and be selected by other consequences to serve an entirely different social function. Further, concepts such as empathy, projection, symbolic aggression, and taking another's perspective could all be traced to the combination and selection of repertoires by social contingencies that could be demonstrated in the pigeon (Andronis, 1987; Andronis, Layng, & Goldiamond, 1997). This brought new insights to understanding issues of symptom choice and the origination of disturbing patterns from nondisturbing components, including diathesis stress models (see, Zubin & Spring, 1977). Clinical practice informed laboratory investigation, and laboratory research, in turn, helped to improve clinical practice.

In 1984, Goldiamond published his last clinical paper that, in greater detail and with more refinement, described his nonlinear analysis and systemic approach. Other papers were published, including one by his students that described their work combining Goldiamond's

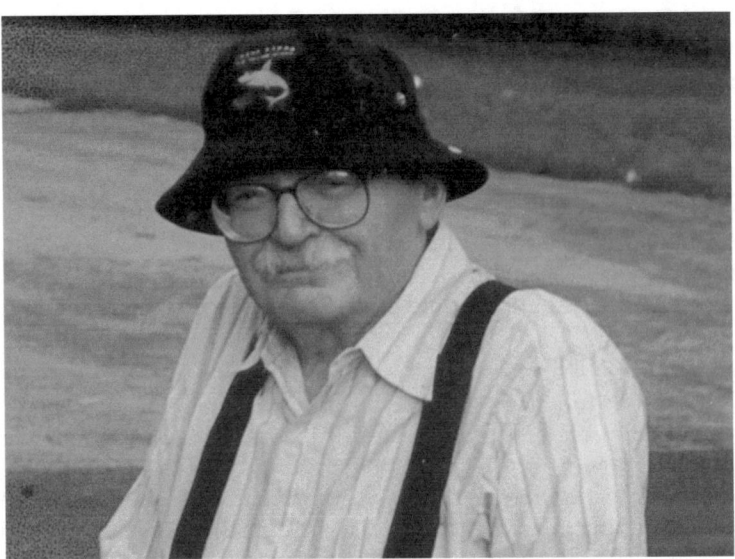

Israel Goldiamond wearing his "Frank Zappa" fishing cap given to him
by Paul Andronis.

nonlinear analysis with Skinner's (1957) approach to verbal behavior in the treatment of
delusions and hallucinations (Layng & Andronis, 1984). Goldiamond retired in the late
1980s, but did not stop working and refining his approach.

Although there were no longer marathon lab meetings in which both experimental and
clinical work were excitedly described, dissected, and analyzed, Goldiamond continued to
collaborate with his students until his death in 1995. Unfortunately, after his death, countless
files, case analyses, intervention details, and data sheets from carefully controlled research
were destroyed, in accord with the privacy policy of the University of Chicago. Nevertheless,
the results of Goldiamond's journey can provide the clinical behavior analyst with extraordinary research and treatment opportunities that may greatly broaden our knowledge of
how selection by consequences can explain complex behavior, emotions, and thought. To
this end, his students have continued to refine and extend both his nonlinear analysis and
his analysis of emotions and emotional behavior. This work is the subject of a larger work
in preparation.

CONCLUSION

Sigrid Glenn (2002) in a retrospective commentary on Goldiamond's constructional approach
eloquently observed,

> In reading again Israel Goldiamond's "Toward a Constructional Approach to Social Problems,"
> I am reminded anew of the scope and power of the work of this great behavior analyst. … But
> most interesting, certainly to the clinician, is the reader's sense of being in the "presence" of a
> truly great clinician. The subtlety and sensitivity, the humor and the understanding, are omni-
> present in the details of treatment that Goldiamond describes. It is interesting that we are able
> to detect that he fully understood and cared about the clients with whom he worked, while he
> consistently described his observations and tactics in scientific terms (with a few apologies for
> everyday language use). (p. 202)

Over many years, Goldiamond and his students helped hundreds of patients. A wide range of conditions were treated including stuttering, obsessive compulsive disorders, panic disorders, eating disorders, phobias, schizophrenia and related diagnoses, borderline syndrome, depression, anxiety, catatonia, drug addiction, posttraumatic stress disorder, brain injury, marital and family problems, and many others. In each case, the disturbing patterns were shown to be sensible outcomes of their nonlinear consequential contingencies, as was the rich and very productive thinking of Israel Goldiamond.

NOTES

It has been over 10 years since the death of Israel Goldiamond. Unfortunately, references to his work are rare. This would not be such a concern if his work was not of such importance to behavior analysis as a field and clinical behavior analysis as a profession. Part of the reason for this lies in the non-behavior-analytic publications in which much of the work appeared, and part lies in the complexity of the work itself. Goldiamond was one of the earliest advocates of a functional analytic approach to behavior. Indeed, his 1967 textbook, which was recently published in slightly edited and revised form (2004, Andronis, Ed.) by the Cambridge Center for Behavioral Studies was titled *The Functional Analysis of Behavior*. He later extended that work to a very sophisticated nonlinear functional analysis that provides a unique perspective on understanding complex behavior, and particularly behavior of clinical significance. Equipped with this analysis, behavior analysts can understand, treat, and make sense of the seemingly irrational or maladaptive patterns observed in the clinic without resort to hypothetical mediating variables such as emotional avoidance, governance by self-generating misrules, or defective cognitions. This paper is an attempt to provide the foundation of the approach through the personal journey of Israel Goldiamond. It is necessarily circumspect, leaving out much of his work and interests in favor of emphasizing that which is most relevant to the current topic. (For a broader treatment of Goldiamond's impact on behavior analysis, see Gimenez, Layng, & Andronis, 2003.)

This is the scientific journey that led one of behavior analysis' greatest thinkers to his many discoveries, and to his scientifically derived and compassionate constructional approach to human problems based on a nonlinear contingency analysis. This nonlinear analysis provides the basis for sophisticated topical and systemic interpersonal, social, and societal interventions.

I thank Paul Andronis, Lincoln Gimenes, Russell Layng, Zachary Layng, Marta Leon, Charles Merbitz, Edward Morris, Joanne Robbins, Jesús Rosales-Ruiz, Melinda Sota, and Janet Twyman for their encouragement and very helpful comments.

Address correspondence to the author at 4705 S. Dakota St., Seattle, Washington 98118 (e-mail: joe@headsprout. com).

1   A graduate student somehow lost the data for all but one of the subjects run by Goldiamond and Dyrud, so the results of these experiments would never be published. Still, they had had their effect on Goldiamond, which is why the description is included here. Goldiamond was fond of describing the precise details of these experiments, and there were some attempts to replicate them in nonpsychatric settings, but they were never completed.

2   Several papers from this period describe applications of this emerging nonlinear approach; see for example, Goldiamond (1970, 1974a), Layng, Merley, Cohen, Andronis, and Layng (1976), and Merley and Layng (1976). Goldiamond encouraged his students to investigate other related behavior-analytic work from the period that could be considered to fall into a subcategory of his nonlinear formulation such as research into the matching law (Herrnstein, 1961) and its derivations (Baum, 1974). Goldiamond also encouraged his students to read work from other disciplines that analyzed complex nonlinear relations; these included sociology's exchange theory (Homans, 1958), anthropology's transactionalism (Barth, 1969), economics' game theory (von Neuman & Morgenstern, 1944), and psychology's decision theory (Lee, 1973).

3   Just as nondiscriminative avoidance may seem difficult to understand in the laboratory without postulating escape from increasing anxiety or fear, there is a similar appeal to employing escape from some internal feeling or thought as an explanation for some behaviors observed in the clinic. Both are predictable outcomes of a linear contingency analysis. But if one takes a nonlinear or alternative sets approach and asks, "What happens to the rat if the bar is not pressed?," one soon realizes that all behaviors other than bar pressing are candidates for shock, a form of differential punishment of other behavior (DPO), the converse of differential reinforcement of other behavior (DRO). In DRO, all behaviors other than the target behavior are candidates for reinforcement, and the target behavior decreases. A two-factor account of DRO might suggest that elation may build as the timer times down to consequence delivery, the occurrence of the target behavior interrupts the elation, thereby punishing the target behavior. To bring it into correspondence with more recent approaches, perhaps the target behavior comes to signal a period of no reinforcement, and that signal becomes the punisher. None of these explanations may be required when the pattern is considered to be a function of the joint effect of the consequential arrangement on

all classes of behavior. A nonlinear contingency analysis leaves us with sensible rats: bar pressing yields no shock; doing something else receives shock (DPO); bar pressing yields no food, doing something else receives food (DRO). (For a more technical description of these relations and their relation to other laboratory observations, see Goldiamond, 1975a.)

4   This formulation overlaps with one described by Skinner (1953), which considers emotions as by-products of behaving under certain circumstances, but it differs in its specificity in regard to how changes in emotions precisely describe changes in contingencies, and in the distinction between emotion and emotional behavior.

5   No surveys, emotional indexes, or other mental tests were used. Years of psychophysical research have shown these indicators to be highly unreliable. The reader will recall the correspondence in the survey responses of college students to the survey responses of what pilots felt in combat. Patient verbal behavior can change such that words indicating satisfaction may increase in frequency and come to more closely correspond to survey entries indicating improvement (the score sheet). One form of therapy may be judged more successful than another if it produces more matches to a specified "measurement instrument" than another therapy. Change the score sheet, and the result might reverse. As Goldiamond was fond of saying, "insight is achieved when the patient describes his or her behavior as the therapist would."

REFERENCES

Andronis, P. T. (1987). Spontaneous cooperation between pigeons: An experimental analysis of some determinants of a complex social pattern. *Proceedings of the American Association for the Advancement of Science, 153* (Abstract 607).

Andronis, P. T., Layng, T. V. J., & Goldiamond, I. (1997). Contingency adduction of "symbolic aggression" by pigeons. *The Analysis of Verbal Behavior, 14*, 5–17.

Azrin, N. H., Holz, W., & Goldiamond, I. (1961). Response bias in questionnaire reports. *Journal of Consulting Psychology, 25*, 324–326.

Azrin, N. H., Holz, W., Ulrich, R., & Goldiamond, I. (1961). The control of content of conversation through reinforcement. *Journal of the Experimental Analysis of Behavior, 4*, 25–30.

Azrin, N. H., & Nunn, R. G. (1973). Habit reversal: A method of eliminating nervous habits and tics. *Behavior Research & Therapy, 11*, 619–628.

Barth, F. (1969). *Ethnic groups and boundaries: The social organization of cultural difference.* London: Allen & Unwin.

Baum, W. M. (1974). On two types of deviation from the matching law: Bias and undermatching. *Journal of the Experimental Analysis of Behavior, 22*, 231–242.

Chance, P. (1994). *Learning and behavior* (3rd ed.). Pacific Grove, CA: Brooks/Cole.

Dyrud, J. (1971). Treatment of anxiety states. *Archives of General Psychiatry, 25*, 298–305.

Estes, W. K., & Skinner, B. F. (1941). Some quantitative properties of anxiety. *Journal of Experimental Psychology, 29*, 390–400.

Flanagan, B., Goldiamond, I., & Azrin, N. H. (1958). Operant stuttering: The control of stuttering behavior through response contingent consequences. *Journal of the Experimental Analysis of Behavior, 1*, 173–177.

Flanagan, B., Goldiamond, I., & Azrin, N. H. (1959). Instatement of stuttering in normally fluent individuals through operant procedures. *Science, 130*(3381), 979–981.

Gimenez, L. S., Andronis, P. T., & Goldiamond, I. (1987). Estudo de algumas variaveis de procedimento na defecacao induzida por esquemas de reforcamento [Study of some procedural variables on schedule-induced defecation]. *Psicologia: Teoria e Pesquisa, 3*(2), 104–116.

Gimenez, L. S., Layng, T. V. J., & Andronis, P. T. (2003). Contribuições de Israel Goldiamond para o desenvolvimento da análise do comportamento [Contributions of Israel Goldiamond to the development of the analysis of behavior.] In M. Brando et al. (Eds.), *Sobre comportamento e cognicao* (Vol. 11, pp. 34–46). Santo Andre, Brazil: ESETec Editores Associados.

Glenn, S. S. (2002). Retrospective on Goldiamond's "Toward a Constructional Approach to Social Problems." *Behavior and Social Issues, 11*(2), 202–203.

Goldiamond, I. (1958). Indicators of perception: I. Subliminal perception, subception, unconscious perception: An analysis in terms of psychophysical indicator methodology. *Psychological Bulletin, 55*, 373–411.

Goldiamond, I. (1959). The hysteria over subliminal advertising as a misunderstanding of science. *American Psychologist, 14*, 598–599.

Goldiamond, I. (1962). Perception. In A. J. Bachrach (Ed.), *The experimental foundations of clinical psychology* (pp. 280–340). New York: Basic Books.

Goldiamond, I. (1964a). A research and demonstration procedure in stimulus control, abstraction, and environmental programming. *Journal of the Experimental Analysis of Behavior, 7*, 216.

Goldiamond, I. (1964b). Response bias in perceptual communication. In *Disorders of communication. Research Publications of the Association for Research in Nervous and Mental Diseases, 42*, chapter 23.

Goldiamond, I. (1965a). Self-control procedures in personal behavior problems. *Psychological Reports, 17,* 851–868. Monograph Supplement 3-V 17. (Reprinted in R. W. Ulrich, T. J. Stachnik, & J. H. Mabry (Eds.), *The control of human behavior* (pp. 115–122). Chicago: Scott Foresman.)

Goldiamond, I. (1965b). Stuttering and fluency as manipulatable operant response classes. In L. Krasner & L. P. Ullman (Eds.), *Research in behavior modification* (pp. 106–156). New York: Holt, Rinehart, & Winston.

Goldiamond, I. (1966). Perception, language, and conceptualization rules. In B. Kleinmuntz (Ed.), *Problem solving* (pp. 183–224). New York: Wiley.

Goldiamond, I. (1968). Moral behavior: A functional analysis. *Psychology Today, 2*(9), 31–34, 69–70.

Goldiamond, I. (1969). Applications of operant conditioning. In C. A. Thomas (Ed.), *Current trends in army medical service psychology* (pp. 198–231). Aurora, CO: Department of the Army, Fitzsimmons General Hospital.

Goldiamond, I. (1970). Human control over human behavior. In M. Wertheimer (Ed.), *Confrontation: Psychology and the problems of today* (pp. 254–406). Glenview, IL: Scott Foresman.

Goldiamond, I. (1974a). A diary of self-modification. *Psychology Today, 11,* 95–102.

Goldiamond, I. (1974b). Toward a constructional approach to social problems: Ethical and constitutional issues raised by applied behavior analysis. *Behaviorism, 2,* 1–84.

Goldiamond, I. (1975a). Alternative sets as a framework for behavioral formulations and research. *Behaviorism, 3,* 49–85.

Goldiamond, I. (1975b). A constructional approach to self control. In A. Schwartz & I. Goldiamond (Eds.), *Social casework: A behavioral approach* (pp. 67–130). New York: Columbia University.

Goldiamond, I. (1975c). Singling out behavior modification for legal regulation: Some effects on patient care, psychotherapy, and research in general. *Arizona Law Review, 17,* 105–126.

Goldiamond, I. (1976a). Protection of human subjects and patients: A social contingency analysis of distinctions between research and practice, and its implications. *Behaviorism, 4*(1), 1–41.

Goldiamond, I. (1976b). Singling out self-administered behavior therapies for professional overview. *American Psychologist, 31,* 142–147.

Goldiamond, I. (1977). Insider-outsider problems: A constructional approach. *Rehabilitation Psychology, 22,* 103–116.

Goldiamond, I. (1978). *A programming contingency analysis of mental health* (MABA Presidential Speech, revised and expanded 1983). Israel Goldiamond Papers, Accession No. 2005-59, University of Chicago Library Special Collections Research Center Archives and Manuscripts.

Goldiamond, I. (1979a). Behavioral approaches and liaison psychiatry. *Psychiatric Clinics of North America, 2,* 379–401.

Goldiamond, I. (1979b). *Emotions and emotional behavior: A consequential analysis and treatment.* Audiotape, Association for the Advancement of Behavior Therapy. New York: BMA Audio Cassettes Publisher.

Goldiamond, I. (1984). Training parents and ethicists in nonlinear behavior analysis. In R. F. Dangel & R. A. Polster (Eds.), *Parent training: Foundations of research and practice* (pp. 504–546). New York: Guilford.

Goldiamond, I., Atkinson, C. J., & Bilger, R.C. (1962). Stabilization of behavior under prolonged exposure to delayed auditory feedback. *Science, 135,* 437–438.

Goldiamond, I., & Dyrud, J. E. (1968). Some applications and implications of behavioral analysis for psychotherapy. In J. M. Shlien (Ed.), *Research in psychotherapy* (Vol. 3, pp. 54–89). Washington, DC: American Psychological Association.

Goldiamond, I., Dyrud, J., & Miller, M. (1965). Practice as research in professional psychology. *Canadian Psychologist, 6,* 110–128.

Goldiamond, I., & Flanagan, B. (1959). Operant stuttering: The use of delayed feedback as aversive stimulus in the operant control of stuttering. *Journal of the American Speech and Hearing Association, 1,* 93.

Goldiamond, I., & Hawkins, W. F. (1958). Vexierversuch: The log relationship between word-frequency and recognition obtained in the absence of stimulus words. *Journal of Experimental Psychology, 56,* 457–463.

Goldiamond, I., & Malpass, L. F. (1961). Locus of hypnotically induced changes in color vision responses. *Journal of the Optical Society of America,* 1117–1121.

Goldiamond, I., & Schwartz, A. (1975). The Smith case. In A. Schwartz & I. Goldiamond (Eds.), *Social casework: A behavioral approach* (pp. 131–192). New York: Columbia University.

Goldiamond, I., & Thompson, D. (2004). The blue books: Goldiamond & Thompson's the functional analysis of behavior, P. T. Andronis (Ed.). Cambridge, MA: Cambridge Center for Behavioral Studies. (Original work published 1967.)

Herrnstein, R. J. (1961). Relative and absolute strength of response as a function of frequency of reinforcement. *Journal of the Experimental Analysis of Behavior, 4,* 267–272.

Holz, W., & Azrin, N. (1961). Discriminative properties of punishment. *Journal of the Experimental Analysis of Behavior, 4,* 225–232.

Homans, G. C. (1958). Social behavior as exchange. *The American Journal of Sociology, 63,* 597–606.

Isaacs, W., Thomas, J., & Goldiamond, I. (1960). Application of operant conditioning procedures to reinstate verbal behavior in psychotics. *Journal of Speech and Hearing Disorders, 25,* 8–12.

Keller, F. S., & Schoenfeld, W. N. (1960). *Principles of psychology: A systematic text in the science of behavior.* Cambridge, MA: B.F. Skinner Foundation. (Original work published 1950.)

Layng, T. V. J. (1995). Causation and complexity: Old lessons new crusades. *Journal of Behavior Therapy and Experimental Psychiatry, 26*, 249–258.

Layng, T. V. J. (2006). Emotions and emotional behavior: A constructional approach to understanding some social benefits of aggression. *Brazilian Journal of Behavior Analysis, 2*(2), 155–170.

Layng, T. V. J., & Andronis, P. T. (1984). Toward a functional analysis of delusional speech and hallucinatory behavior. *The Behavior Analyst, 7*, 139–156.

Layng, T. V. J., Andronis, P. T., & Goldiamond, I. (1999). Animal models of psychopathology: The establishment, maintenance, attenuation, and persistence of head banging by pigeons. *Journal of Behavior Therapy and Experimental Psychiatry, 30*, 45–61.

Layng, T. V. J., Merley, S., Cohen, J., Andronis, P. T., & Layng, M. (1976). *Programmed instruction, self-control, and in-patient psychiatry.* Educational Resource Clearinghouse (ERIC), Document Listing No. 142 886.

Lee, W. (1971). *Decision theory and human behavior.* New York: Wiley.

Merley, S., & Layng, T. V. J. (1976). In-patient psychiatry and programed instruction: Application and research in constructional theory. *Improving Human Performance Quarterly, 5*, 35–46.

Rayfield, F., Segal, M., & Goldiamond, I. (1982). Schedule-induced defecation. *Journal of the Experimental Analysis of Behavior, 38*, 19–34.

Sidman, M. (1958). By-products of aversive control. *Journal of the Experimental Analysis of Behavior, 1*, 265–280.

Sidman, M. (1960). Normal sources of pathological behavior. *Science, 132*, 61–68.

Skinner, B. F. (1953). *Science and human behavior.* New York: Free Press.

Skinner, B. F. (1957). *Verbal behavior.* Englewood Cliffs, NJ: Prentice Hall.

Skinner, B. F. (1966). An operant analysis of problem solving. In B. Kleinmuntz (Ed.), *Problem solving: Research, method and theory* (pp. 225–257). New York: Wiley. (Reprinted in *Contingencies of reinforcement: A theoretical analysis.* New York: Appleton Century-Crofts, 1969.)

Skinner, B. F. (1977). The force of coincidence. *Humanist, 31*(3), 10–11.

Travis, M. (1982). *Matching client entry repertoires and professional programming repertoires in a nutrition program.* Unpublished doctoral dissertation, University of Chicago.

Von Neumann, J., & Morgenstern, O. (1944). *Theory of games and economic behavior.* Princeton, NJ: Princeton University Press.

Zubin, J., & Spring, B. (1977). Vulnerability: A new view of schizophrenia. *Journal of Abnormal Psychology, 86*, 103–126.

Index

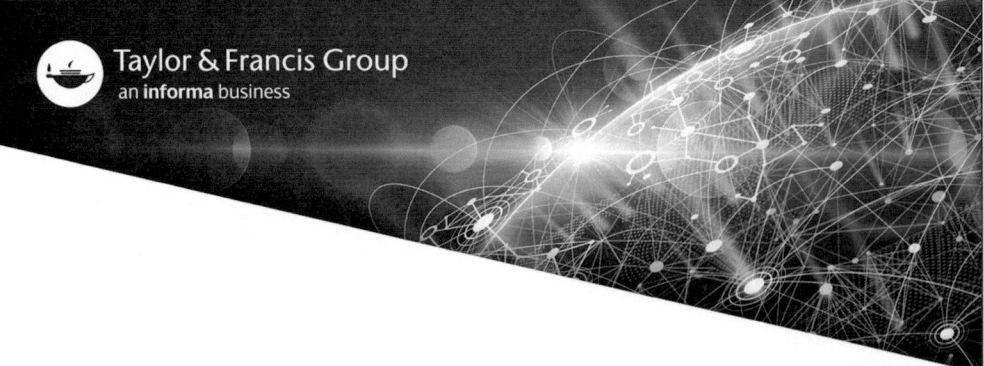
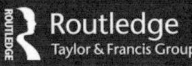
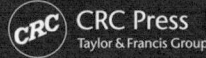